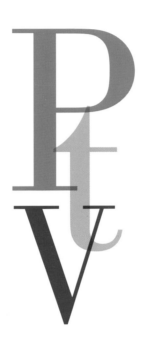

PART-TIME VEGETARIAN
SMOOTHIES AND JUICES

Boost your immune system and
increase your energy with
a flexitarian diet

Tina Haupert

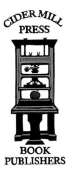

CIDER MILL PRESS

BOOK PUBLISHERS

Kennebunkport, Maine

Contents

To my husband, Mal, for his support, love, patience, humor, and constant willingness to taste-test smoothies and juices. I love you.

Introduction

In recent years, thanks to breakthrough studies on food and nutrition as well as eye-opening documentaries and publications, we've seen an increase in vegan dieting, which has skyrocketed blender and juicer sales. A whole-food, plant-based diet is proving to be one of the best routes to optimal health and nutrition.

If a plant-based diet is so healthy, why aren't more people getting on board? For a lot of people, the thought of eliminating meat and dairy from their diet can be overwhelming and a bit daunting. This book provides to be a middle ground for those looking to decrease their intake of animal products by filling up on vegetarian or even vegan smoothies and juices during the day, while not eliminating the foods they love so much from their dinner plates.

Drinking smoothies and freshly pressed juice is a great way to support this "flexitarian" lifestyle while ensuring that you're getting a nutrient-dense diet by making it easy to consume the recommended daily requirement for fruits and vegetables. It's amazing how many fruits and vegetables you can combine in one glass! And, of course, a diet packed full of nutrients is essential to a healthy body and your well-being.

As you'll quickly discover, drinking your fruits and veggies is a convenient way for you

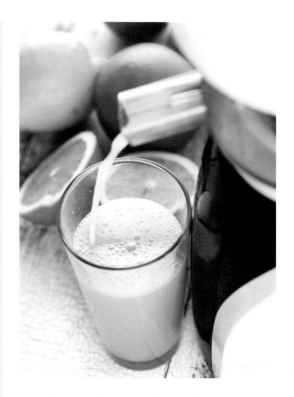

to add more fresh produce and nutrients to your diet. Both smoothies and juice help you fill the nutritional gaps when your diet falls short, because they make it possible to "eat the rainbow." Plus, you might even find yourself enjoying smoothies and juice with ingredients you might not have liked before! And, of course, this is a much healthier way to eat than loading melted cheese on your broccoli florets, right?

I hope this book helps you to get more fruits and vegetables in your diet through delicious drinks you'll come to crave again and again.

Tina Haupert

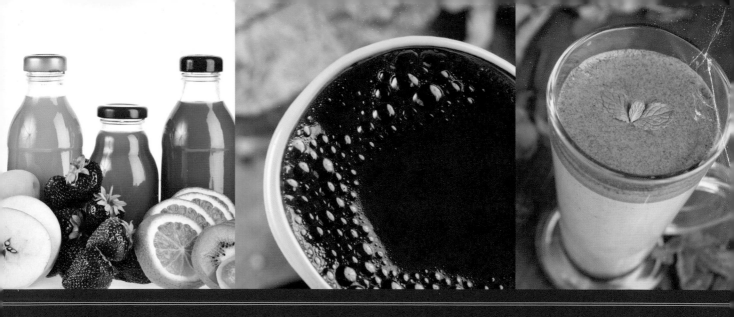

Chapter 1

Getting Started

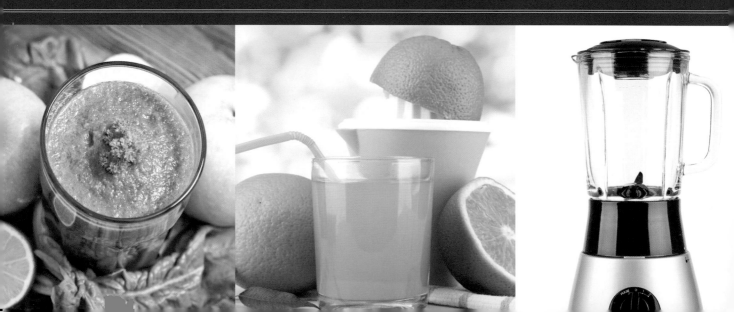

*I*t's important to have the right tools when it comes to making healthful smoothies and juice. In this first chapter, you'll learn about what to look for in a blender and a juicer, selecting the ingredients, and best practices for producing the highest-quality smoothies and juice.

It might seem like there's a lot to know, but the best way to make delicious-tasting smoothies and juice is to experiment with your favorite flavors and ingredients. There's no right or wrong way to make them. As long as you're including plenty of fruits, veggies, and other nutrient-rich ingredients, your overall health and wellness will benefit.

Choosing a Blender

There are two main types of blenders: countertop and handheld/immersion blenders. Countertop blenders tend to be larger and more powerful, which makes them a great option for smoothies, especially when it comes to blending a variety of different ingredients at once. Although handheld/immersion blenders are also handy for making smoothies, they don't have the same blending powers since they need to be held and submerged in the beverage that you are preparing. They're typically better for blending simple smoothies and protein shakes than those made with ice cubes and frozen fruits and vegetables.

When it comes to pulverizing frozen fruit and crushing ice in smoothies, you want to use a heavy-duty and powerful machine. Blenders typically range from 300 to more than 1,200 watts. In general, higher wattage translates to better performance, but a blender with 500 watts might just be what you're looking for. But if you're going to want to crush ice—and nearly everyone does—you'll want a model with high-speed blades.

More speeds on a blender do not necessarily make it a better piece of equipment. Let's say you have 16 speeds. It might seem like a great feature, but it's hard to distinguish between one from another. Instead, choose a blender with fewer speed settings, but one with at

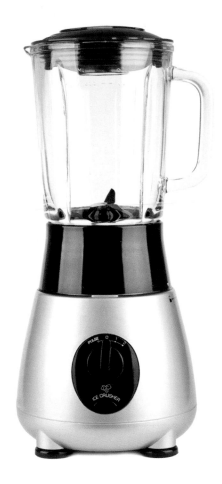

least three options: low, high, and pulse. That way, you have the option of blending your smoothies and their specific ingredients at different speeds as needed.

Blender containers are made of glass, plastic, or stainless steel and hold about 4 to 8 cups. A lot of people prefer glass containers because they're stable and easy to clean. But they're also heavier and typically more expensive. Plastic is lighter and easy to clean. However, plastic can scratch and can absorb smells. Stainless steel sounds fancy, but you can't see how the blending is going inside.

Whatever blender you decide to purchase, make sure it fits both your lifestyle and budget. Size is particularly important. Ask yourself: Where will you keep the blender? Will it live on your countertop, or do you have storage space for it? Will you make smoothies for your spouse or children or just yourself? Do you plan to make smoothies on a daily basis? These questions will help you decide whether a full-size or handheld blender makes the most sense for you.

Smoothie Tips & Notes

* For the most part, the non-dairy milk selections in this book can be used interchangeably or replaced with cow's milk. (Just avoid mixing cow's milk and citrus ingredients.) The suggested variety for each recipe produce the results I like best, but feel free to experiment. For example, if you're not a fan of soymilk, try almond milk, hemp milk, or cow's milk (if you don't follow a vegan diet) instead, in the same amount. The same goes for yogurt; non-dairy varieties made with almond milk, soymilk, or coconut milk can be used instead. Likewise, protein powder comes in both vegan and non-vegan varieties.

* Many smoothie recipes in this book include honey as a sweetener. If you abide by a strict vegan diet, feel free to substitute agave nectar, maple syrup, coconut nectar, or another vegan sweetener.

* Use fresh, ripe, organic fruits, vegetables, and other ingredients for best results—that is, health benefits, nutrients, and taste.

* Wash and (if necessary) cut all fruits and vegetables before putting them into the blender. If there are any bruised or damaged parts, remove them before blending.

* Ready-frozen fruit is a great option for smoothies since it's just as nutritious as fresh and typically more affordable and convenient. It's also great for out-of-season produce—you can have berry smoothies in the winter! You can either defrost frozen produce prior to use or use it frozen. Using frozen produce adds a rich texture and flavor since ice isn't typically needed.

* If you have about-to-spoil fresh produce on hand, save it for a future smoothies by freezing it. Simply peel (if necessary) and slice it before placing it in a Ziplock bag in the freezer. Same goes for extra yogurt; pour into an ice cube tray and freeze. When the time comes, just pop out a few cubes and toss them in your blender!

* When freezing bananas, be sure to peel them *before* you put them in the freezer.

* For the most part, the non-dairy milk selections in this book can be used interchangeably. The suggested variety for each recipe will produce the best results, but feel free to use your favorite kind. For example, if you're not a fan of soymilk, try almond,

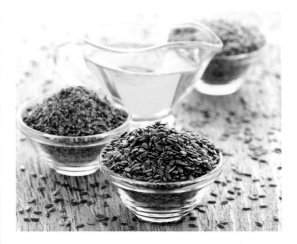

coconut, or hemp milk instead in the same amount. Same goes for non-dairy, vegan yogurt (i.e., those made with almond milk, soymilk, coconut milk, etc.). These varieties can be used interchangeably.

* Superfood ingredients, such as chia seeds, wheatgrass, and flaxseed, can easily be added to all of the smoothies in this book. Some recipes include optional suggestions, but feel free to incorporate these nutrient-dense add-ins to any and all of the smoothies!

* Since this book is based upon a "flexitarian" diet, chocolate-flavored almond and soy milk as well as dark chocolate are added to some of the recipes. These products are not typically vegan foods, so feel free to substitute carob chips or a vegan chocolate products in the recipes as needed.

* Unless otherwise noted, the recipes in this book produce approximately 16-ounce smoothies.

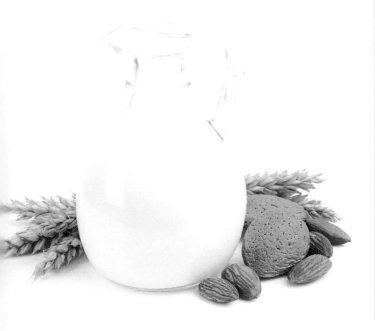

Choosing a Juicer

Electric juicers come in two main types: masticating (also known as cold press because they don't produce heat when they extract the juice) and centrifugal.

A **masticating** juicer works by smashing and crushing fruits and vegetables and then squeezing them through a fine, stainless steel strainer to produce juice. This type of juicer tends to be quieter and extracts more juice and nutrients because it generates less heat and friction. But masticating juicers also tend to be bulkier and more expensive than centrifugal juicers.

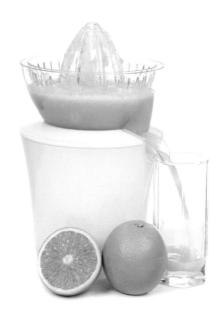

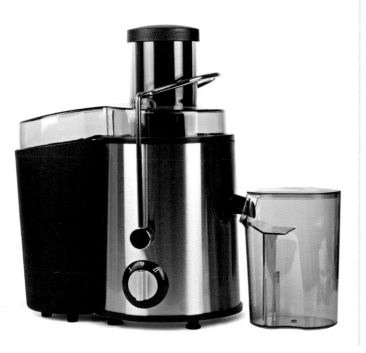

A **centrifugal** juicer has sharp, fast-spinning metal blades that shred the fruits and vegetables and then, using centrifugal force, separate the juice from the pulp, which are then separated into different containers. Some centrifugal juicers have an automatic pulp ejector that sends the pulp into a side container once the juice has been extracted, which makes cleanup easier and faster. Other centrifugal juicers have an extra-wide mouth that allows you to feed larger pieces of fruit and vegetables into the machine, which reduces the time spent cutting up produce to be juiced.

Centrifugal juicers tend to be more popular than masticating juicers because they're (sometimes) faster, easier to use and clean, as well as more affordable. But because the high-speed spinning blades inside the machines create

> *"Don't eat anything your great-great grandmother wouldn't recognize as food."*
>
> —MICHAEL POLLAN

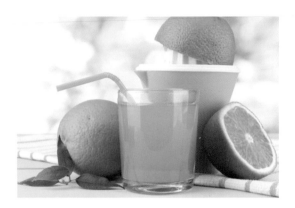

heat, it can break down and destroy some of the enzymes in the fruits and vegetables that you are juicing. The heat also oxides the nutrients, which makes them less nutritious than a masticating (or cold press juicer), which produces no heat.

In the end, it's up to you which kind of juicer fits into your lifestyle and budget. If you're not too picky about getting the most nutrients or don't have a lot of money to spend, the centrifugal juicer might be for you. However, if you want to pack the most nutrients as possible into your body and don't mind spending a few extra bucks, go for the masticating (cold press) juicer.

No matter what you decide, consider the ease of use of the juicer you choose. If it's difficult to use or clean up, you won't use it often, which defeats the purpose of owning a juicer. Request an in-store demonstration, if possible, or watch videos reviews online to see the entire juicing process before purchasing.

Juicing Tips & Notes

* Use fresh, ripe, organic fruits, vegetables, and herbs for best results—that is, health benefits, nutrients, and taste.
* Wash and (if necessary) cut all fruits and vegetables before putting them into the juicer. If there are any bruised or damaged parts, remove them before juicing.
* Remove pits and seeds from fruit before juicing to prevent damaging machine parts.

✱ To help prevent pulp from clogging the machine, alternate soft/wet and hard/leafy produce whenever possible.

✱ Do not pour water, coconut water, or other juices directly into juicer unless specifically directed to do so.

✱ Make only as much juice as you will need and drink it right away because fresh juice will lose flavor and nutrients immediately after juicing.

✱ Be diligent about thoroughly cleaning your juicer after each use. This will not only help keep the machine in good working order but it can also help protect you from food poising caused by the growth of harmful bacteria left on the machine's parts.

✱ If the flavor of a juice is too intense, use water to lessen it. Water also increases the volume of the beverage, so it seems like you're drinking more. And, of course, water hydrates you and gives you a healthy body!

✱ Because juicing machines and fresh produce vary so much and will give you different results, the juice recipes in this book produce one serving, which is equal to approximately 8 ounces of liquid.

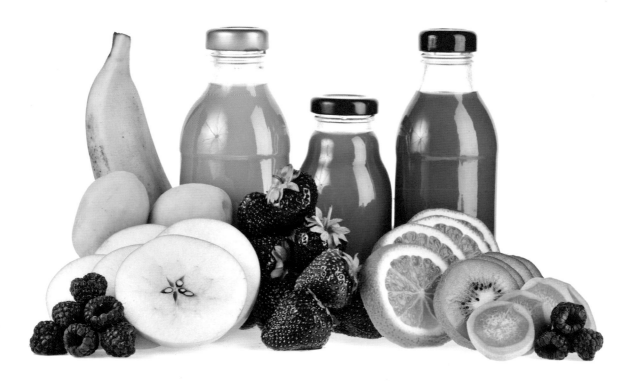

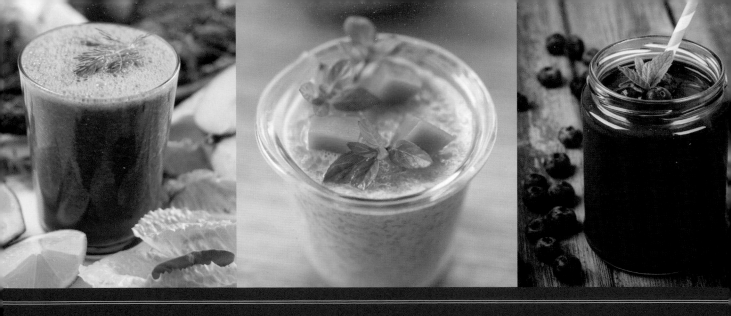

Chapter 2

Breakfast Smoothies

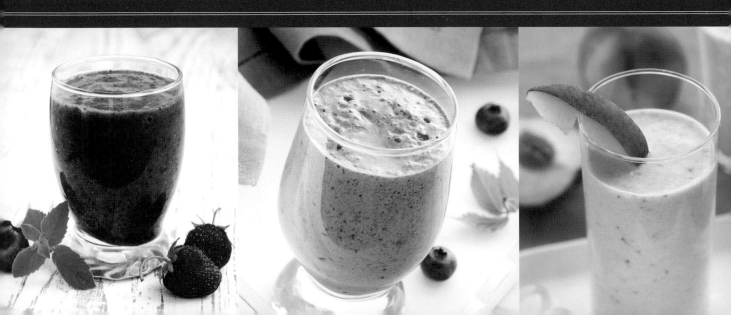

*R*ise and shine! We all know breakfast is the most important meal of the day, so you want to make sure it's both nutritious *and* satisfying. Plus, eating a healthy breakfast sets the tone for your morning, which can help you make smart choices all day long. For these reasons, smoothies are the perfect choice for a quick, nutritious, and delicious breakfast.

The smoothies in this chapter are packed with flavor and nutrients and guaranteed to keep your belly full and happy all morning long. For some added satiety, try a scoop of protein powder in any of these recipes. The protein powder will likely thicken the smoothie, so be ready to add a splash of additional liquid to get it to your preferred consistency.

If you're typically rushed in the morning, know that you can make these smoothies ahead of time. Either add all the ingredients to your blender the night before and store it in the refrigerator overnight to make in the morning, or blend your breakfast smoothie, store it in a travel-friendly container, and then just give it a quick shake up in the morning. Easy as that! You'll have a nutritious and delicious breakfast in no time!

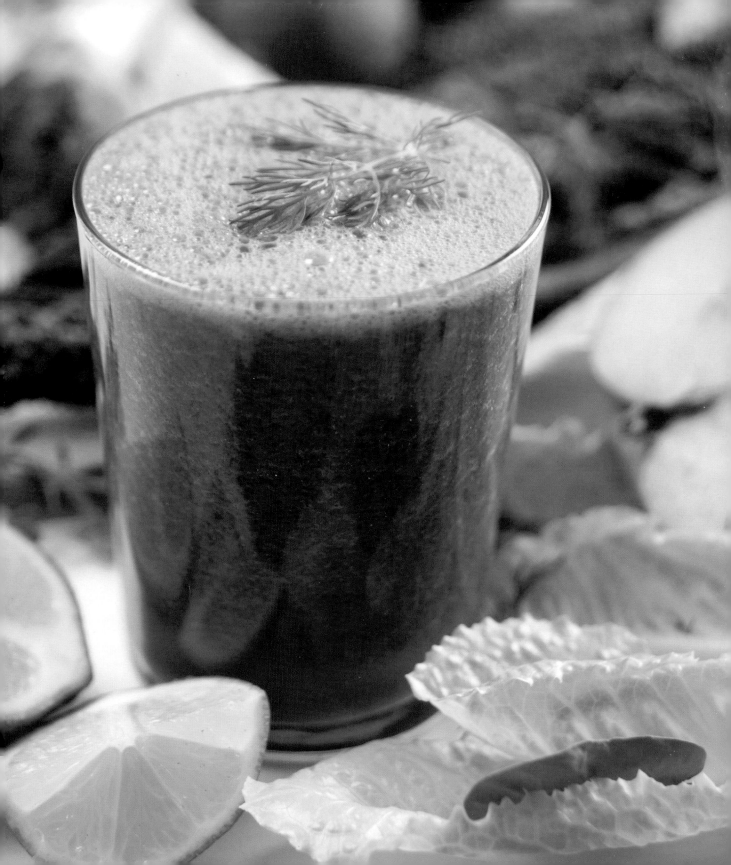

Rise 'N' Shine Smoothie {vegan friendly}

Rise and shine! It's smoothie time! This smoothie will start your day off on the right foot with a whole slew of fresh ingredients and plenty of nutrients. It's tough to have a bad day after drinking down this smoothie!

1 cup fresh spinach, chopped
1 cup fresh romaine, chopped
1 kiwi, peeled and sliced
1 cup apple juice
2 stalks of celery
1 tbsp freshly squeezed lime juice (optional)
4–5 ice cubes

Combine ingredients in a blender until smooth. Pour into a glass and serve immediately.

Try this: For a peppery kick, add a handful of fresh parsley before blending.

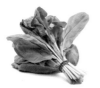   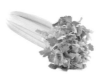

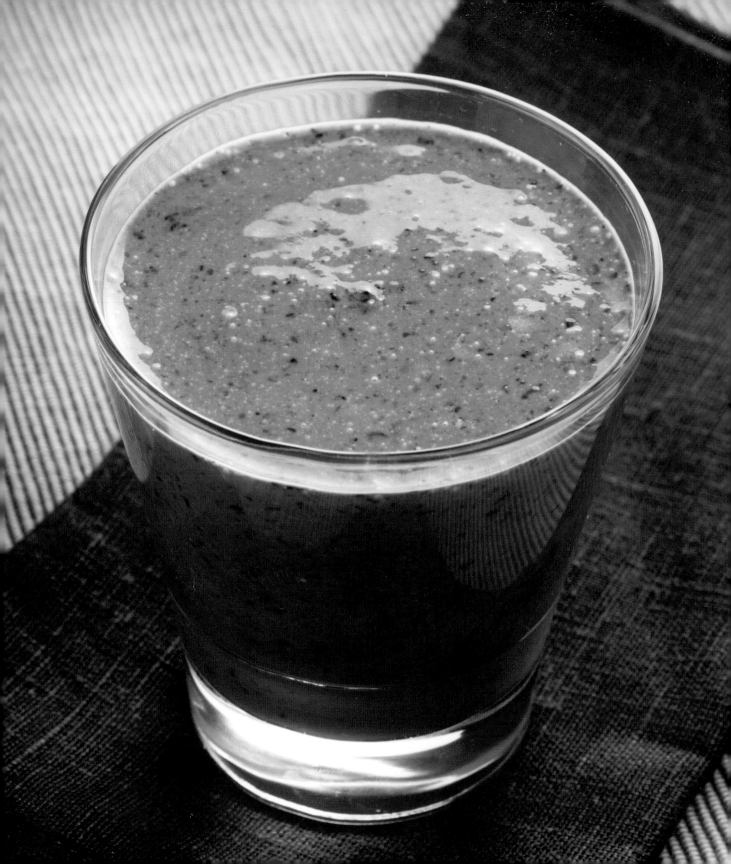

Pearberry Smoothie

One of my favorite ways to start my morning is with fresh fruit, because it sets a healthy tone for the rest of my day. This smoothie will wake you up and getting you going with the sweet flavors of pear, berries, and banana!

½ banana

1 ripe pear, cored and chopped

½ cup frozen mixed berries
(or your choice of berries)

½ cup water

2 tsp honey (or agave nectar) (optional)

Combine ingredients in a blender until smooth. Pour into a glass and enjoy immediately.

> *"There are only ten minutes in the life of a pear when it is perfect to eat."*
>
> —RALPH WALDO EMERSON

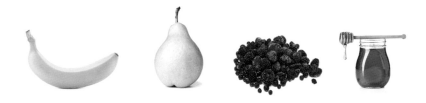

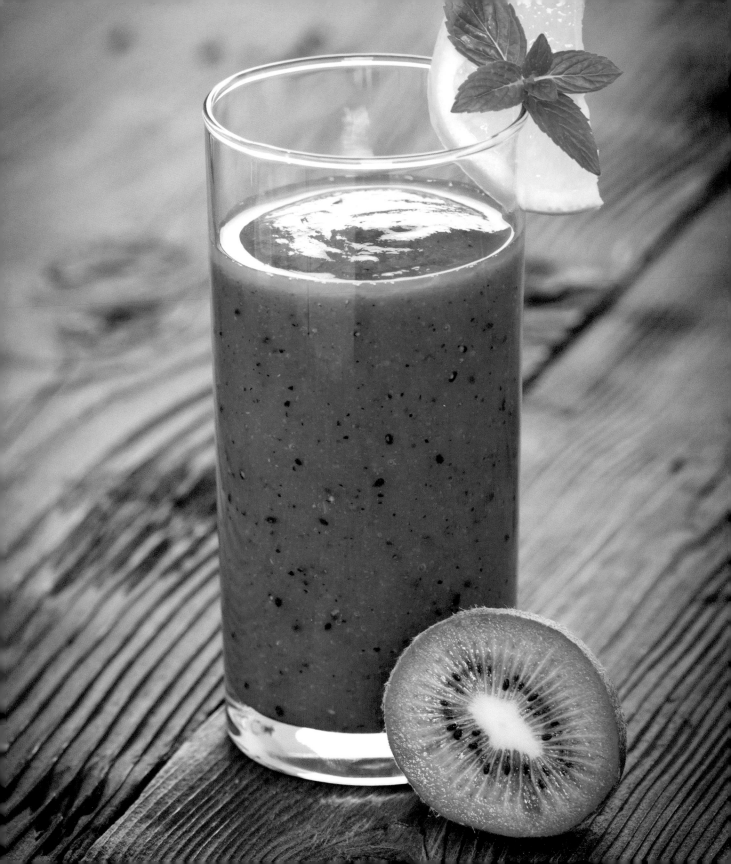

Sunshine Smoothie {vegan friendly}

Here's a smoothie that will supply you with a whole host of vital nutrients while waking you up naturally with bold citrus flavors of orange, lemon, and kiwi. It's like starting your day with a ray of sunshine!

2 cups fresh kale, chopped
2 kiwis, peeled and sliced
1.25 cups orange juice
2 tbsp freshly squeezed lemon juice
4–5 ice cubes

Combine ingredients in a blender until smooth. Pour into a glass and enjoy immediately.

> *"Just living is not enough... one must have sunshine, freedom, and a little flower."*
>
> —Hans Christian Andersen

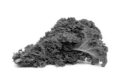 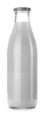

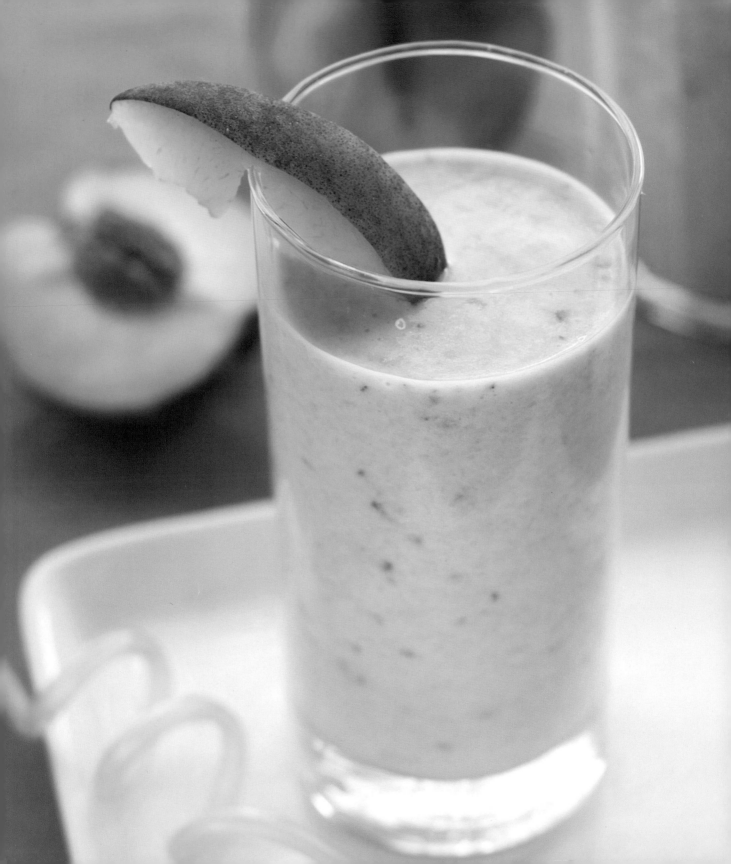

Sweet Citrus Smoothie

If you want to start your day off on the right foot, this smoothie is for you! It's made with a sweet and citrusy mix of flavors to wake you up—taste buds included—and get you moving!

½ banana
½ cup frozen peaches
½ cup frozen raspberries
1 cup orange juice
2 tsp honey (or agave nectar) (optional)

Combine ingredients in a blender until smooth. Pour into a glass and enjoy immediately.

Try this: For a smoothie with zing, add 1 tablespoon of grated ginger before blending.

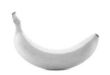 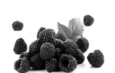

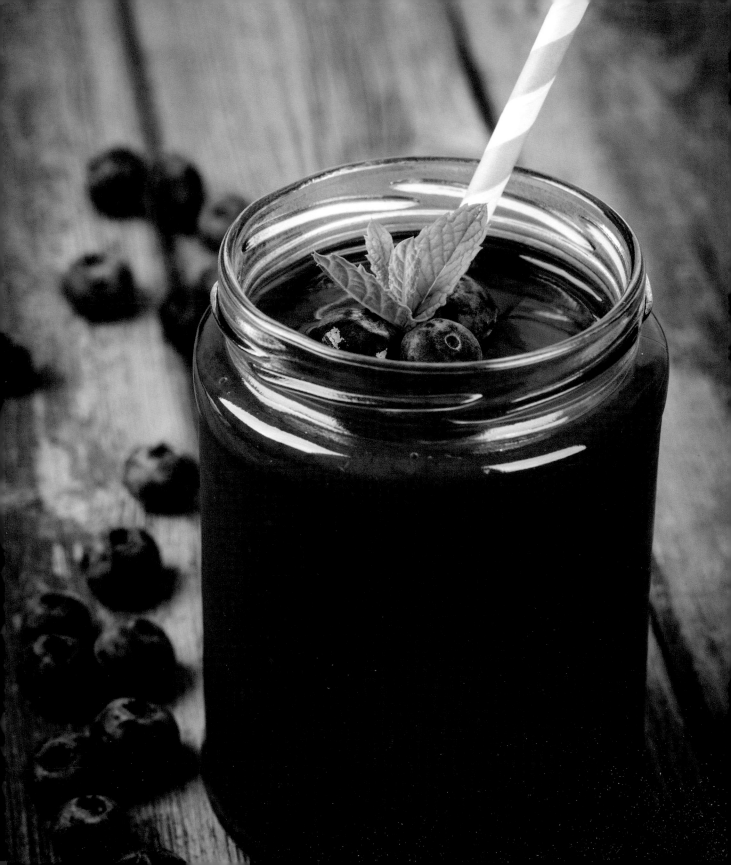

Blueberry Blast

Blast off with this antioxidant-rich smoothie! Blueberries and pomegranate juice will tantalize your taste buds and give you an energy boost right from your very first sip!

1 cup frozen blueberries

½ cup yogurt

½ cup almond milk

¼ cup pomegranate juice

2 tsp honey (or agave nectar)

Combine ingredients in a blender until smooth. Pour into a glass and enjoy immediately.

Try this: For a refreshingly sweet smoothie, add 8–10 fresh mint leaves before blending.

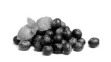 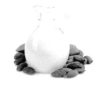

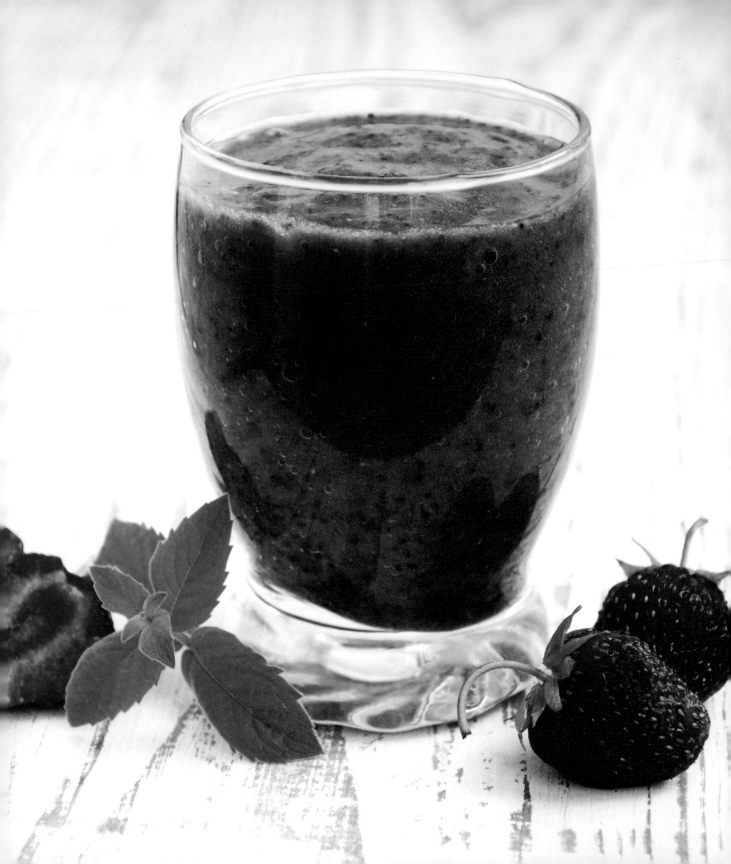

Strawberry-Pomegranate Smoothie

Strawberries and pomegranate combine in this intensely sweet and fresh smoothie. Banana adds a wonderfully thick, creaminess without overpowering the other flavors. This smoothie might just be one of your favorites!

½ banana

1 cup frozen strawberries

1 cup pomegranate juice

2 tsp honey (or agave nectar) (optional)

Combine ingredients in a blender until smooth. Pour into a glass and enjoy immediately.

Strawberries are packed with vitamin C. Just one serving (about eight strawberries) provides more vitamin C than an orange.

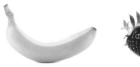

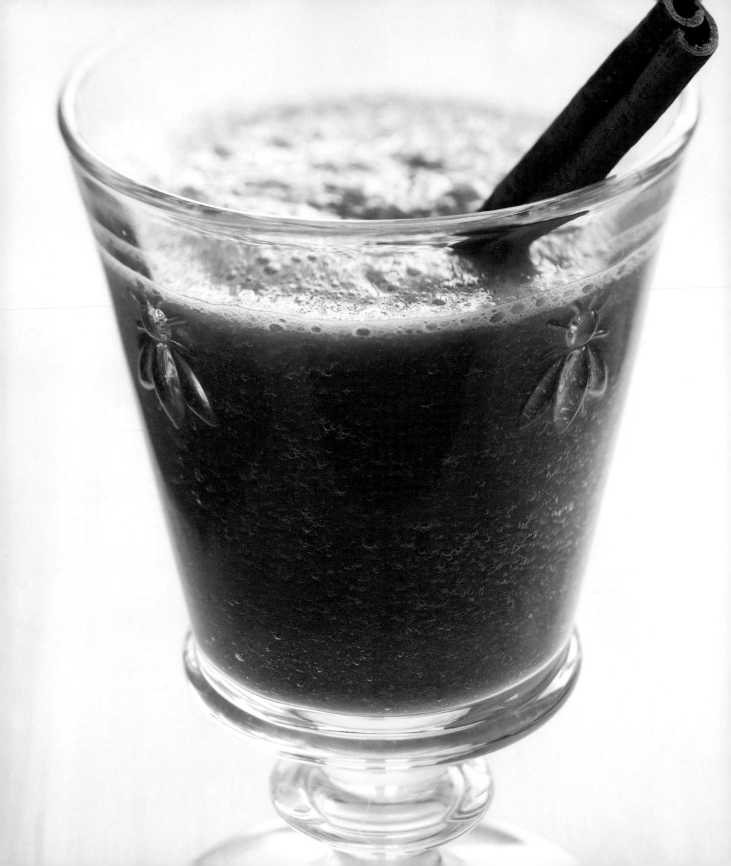

Cinnamon Butternut Smoothie {vegan friendly}

Butternut squash and cinnamon are such a delicious combination, you probably forget they're good for you! This smoothie combines the additional flavors of Medjool dates and vanilla for an even more delightful treat.

½ cup frozen diced butternut squash

½ banana

1.25 cups vanilla almond milk

2 Medjool dates, pitted

½ tsp vanilla extract

1 tsp cinnamon

¼ tsp nutmeg

4–5 ice cubes

Combine ingredients in a blender until smooth. Pour into a glass and enjoy immediately.

Butternut squash is loaded with beta-carotene and vitamin A. It also provides a good amount of vitamin C for a healthy immune system and calcium for strong bones.

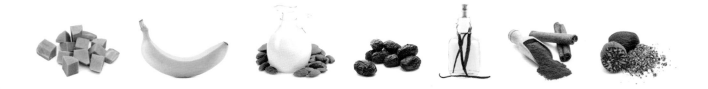

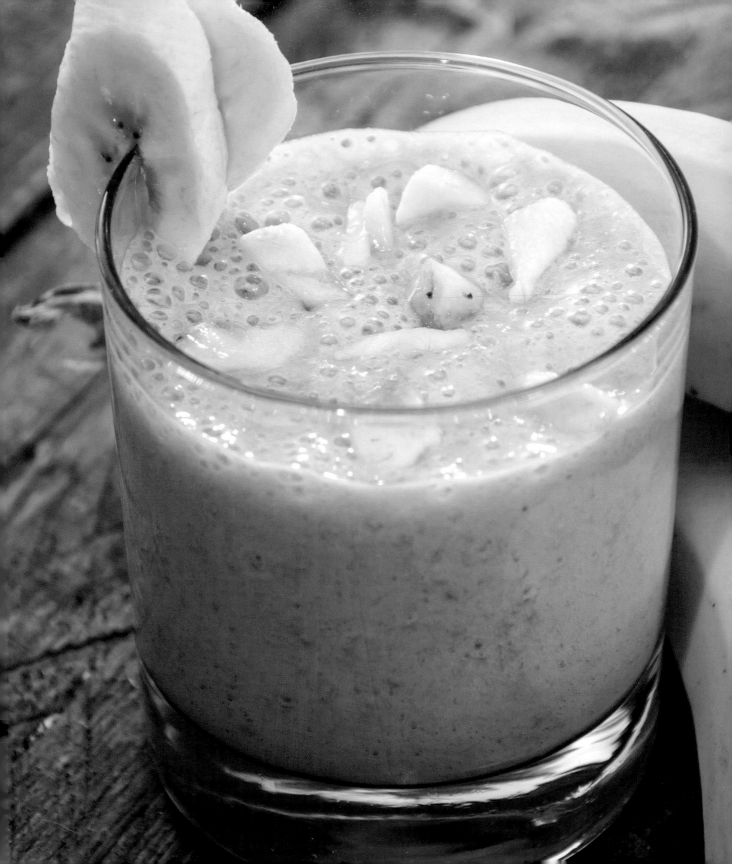

Banana Bread Smoothie

Banana bread for breakfast? Sure, there's nothing better, but who has time to bake first thing in the morning? You can whip up a delicious (and cooler) version in just minutes with this Banana Bread Smoothie!

1 frozen banana

¼ cup rolled oats

1 cup almond milk

1 scoop (20g) your choice of **vanilla** protein powder

1 tbsp ground flaxseed meal

1 tbsp honey (or agave nectar)

Combine ingredients in a blender until smooth. Pour into a glass and enjoy immediately.

Try this: Add **protein** and healthy fats to your Banana Bread Smoothie by adding 2 tablespoons of chopped walnuts before blending.

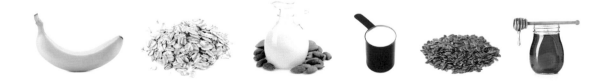

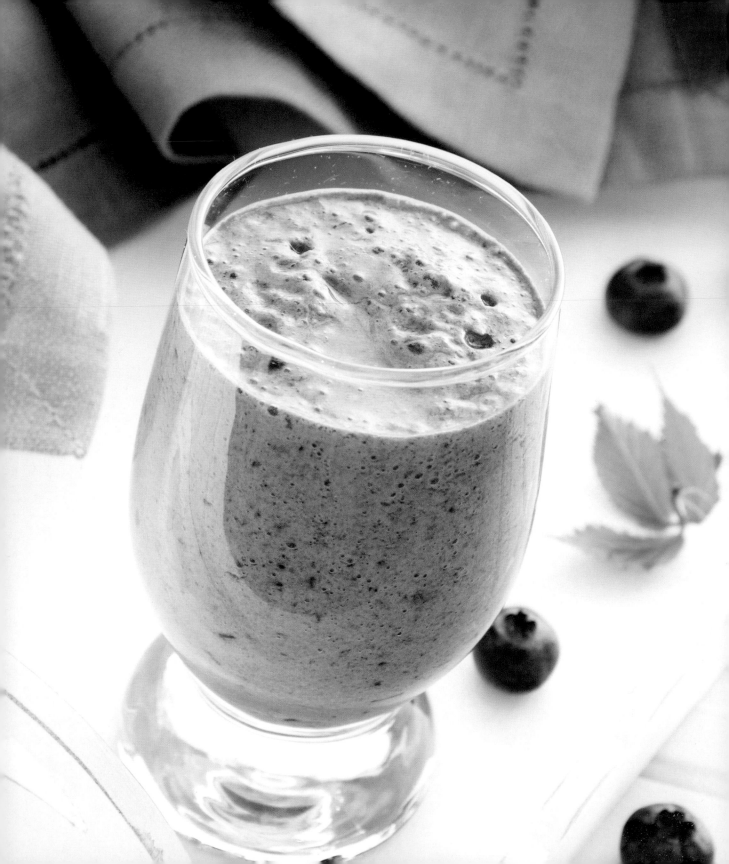

Peanut Butter & Jelly Smoothie

Just about everyone likes peanut butter and jelly sandwiches: They're a quick and easy meal that fills you up and tastes great—and same goes with this smoothie!

1 cup frozen blueberries
1.5 cup almond milk
2-3 tbsp peanut butter
1 tbsp honey (or agave nectar)
¼ tsp vanilla extract
4–5 ice cubes

Combine ingredients in a blender until smooth. Pour into a glass and enjoy immediately.

Who knew? It's estimated that the average American school child will have eaten 1,500 peanut butter and jelly sandwiches before graduation.

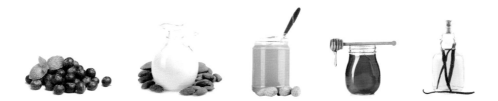

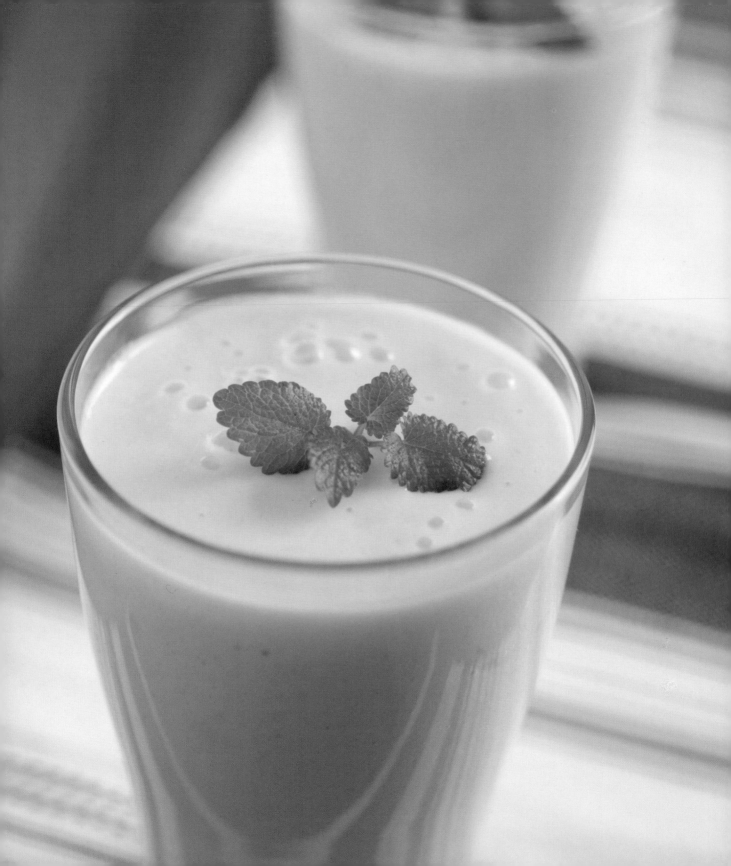

Mighty Mango Smoothie

This Mighty Mango Smoothie will get you moving in the morning. Bold mango and pineapple flavors awaken your senses, and protein powder keeps your stomach satisfied all morning long.

1 cup frozen mango chunks

½ cup frozen pineapple chunks

1 scoop your choice of vanilla protein powder

1 cup almond milk

¾ cup coconut water

Combine ingredients in a blender until smooth. Pour into a glass and enjoy immediately.

Try this: Instead of mango, use 1.5 cups of chunked frozen pineapple for an extra tropical-tasting smoothie.

   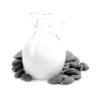

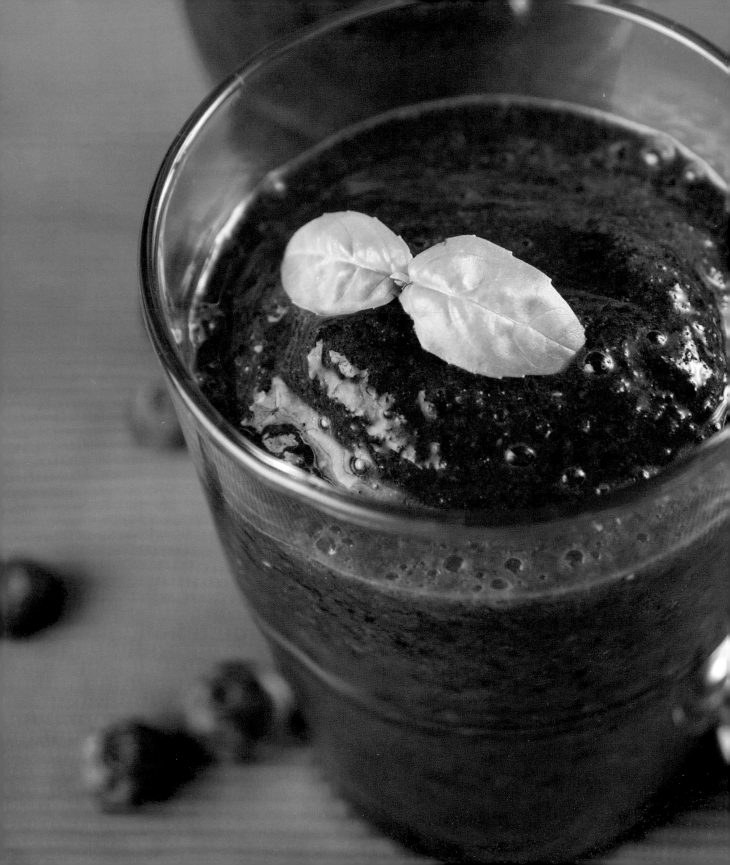

Blueberry-Basil Smoothie {vegan friendly}

From your first sip of this smoothie, the flavors of blueberries, basil, and lemon will give you a natural lift to get you going.

½ cup blueberries

½ frozen banana

1 handful of spinach

1.5 cup almond milk

1 tbsp freshly squeezed lemon juice (optional)

A small handful of fresh basil leaves (approximately 10–12)

Combine ingredients in a blender until smooth. Pour into a glass and enjoy immediately.

Try this: For a minty fresh smoothie, swap out the basil for 8–10 fresh mint leaves before blending.

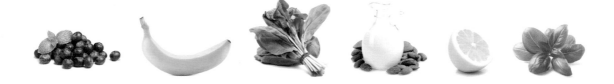

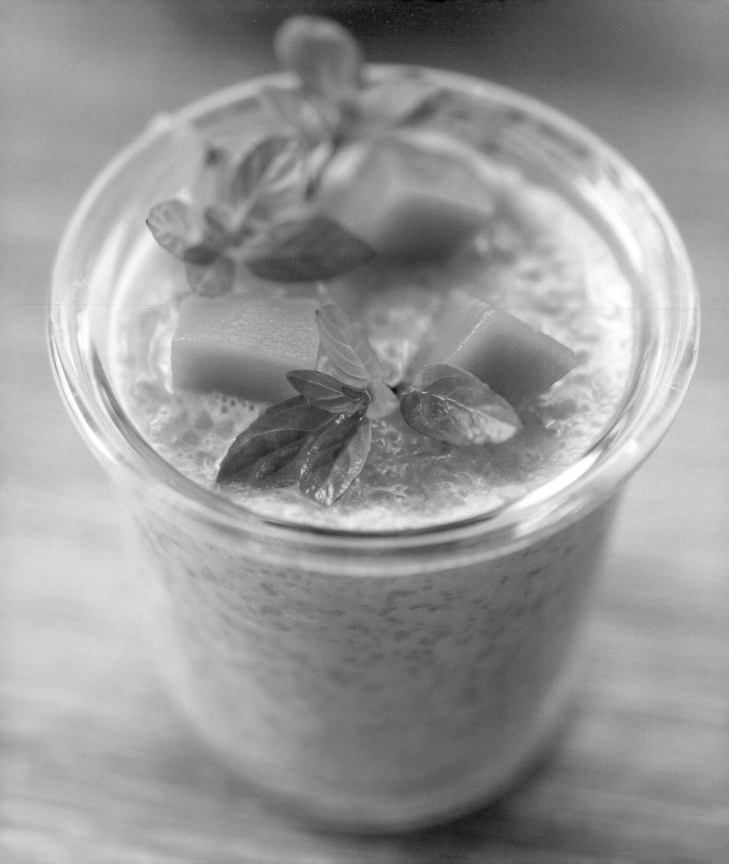

Orange Energizer Smoothie

This bright-orange smoothie will get your attention in more ways than one. Pineapple, pumpkin, orange juice, and freshly grated ginger pack a serious flavor punch.

½ cup frozen pineapple chunks

½ cup pumpkin puree

½ cup yogurt

¾ cup orange juice

1 tbsp maple syrup

½ tsp cinnamon

2 tsp freshly grated ginger

8–10 fresh mint leaves (optional)

4–5 ice cubes

Combine ingredients in a blender until smooth. Pour into a glass, garnish with mint leaves if you'd like, and enjoy immediately.

Pumpkin is an excellent source of the antioxidant beta-carotene. Research shows that people who eat a diet rich in beta-carotene are less likely to develop certain cancers compared to those who don't include beta-carotene–rich foods in their diet.

   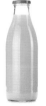

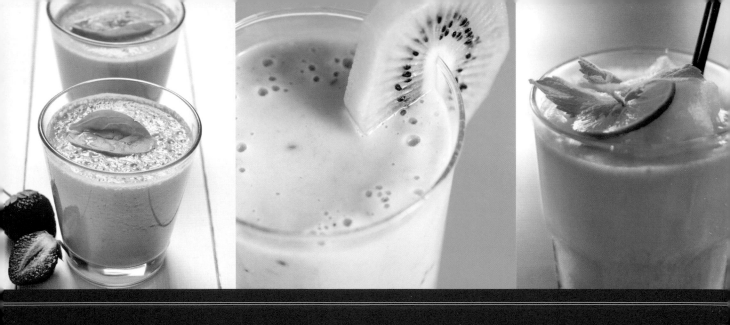

Chapter 3

Green Smoothies

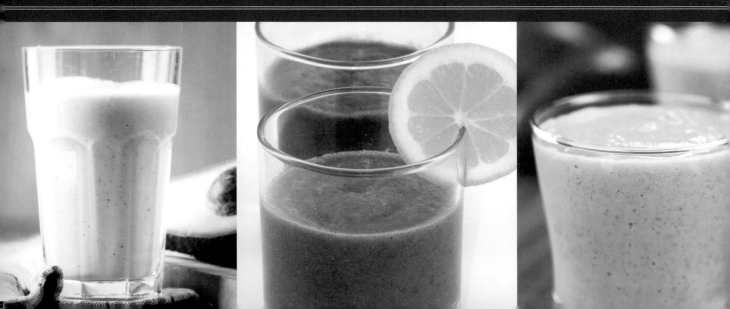

When you're hustling through your day, a green smoothie is a convenient way to get the plant-powered goodness of dark leafy greens in your diet. Just think about: spinach and kale mixed with banana and almond milk—all in one quick, easy meal. It's truly the freshest and fastest way to get nutrient-rich vegetable into your diet.

Vegetables in a smoothie? It might sound a bit odd and perhaps not very appetizing, but you might be surprised how delicious a green smoothie can be. They might even be considered a *treat* by some people. Really!

You will get plenty of vitamins, minerals, fiber, and antioxidants in a single green smoothie. Many of us don't typically eat raw kale, spinach, or parsley on a regular basis—or at least not in the amount called for in a green smoothie. Green smoothies make it really easy for you to get a whole host of vital nutrients into your diet without much effort. And when these leafy greens and other vegetables are combined with sweet fruits, such as bananas, fresh berries, and mango, you won't even taste them. Promise!

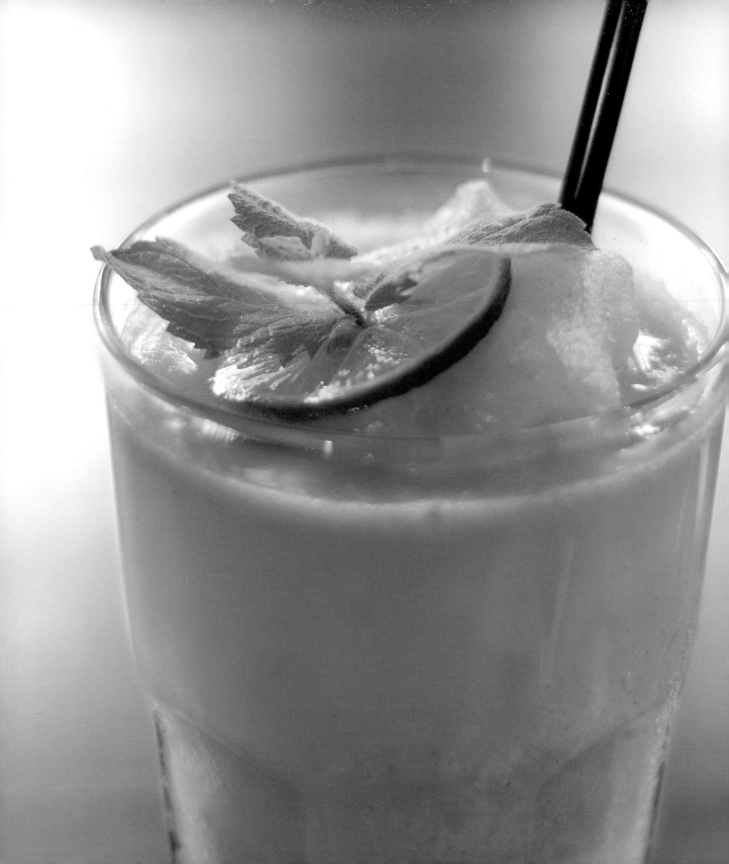

Coconut-Kale Smoothie {vegan friendly}

A taste of the tropics! Loaded with kale, banana, and ground flaxseed, this nutrient-rich smoothie is so delicious and refreshing, you won't even know it's good for you.

1 frozen banana
1 cup frozen chopped kale
1.5 cups coconut milk
1 tbsp ground flaxseed meal
1 tbsp honey (or agave nectar)
¼ tsp coconut extract

Combine ingredients in a blender until smooth. Pour into a glass and serve immediately.

Cruciferous veggies, such as kale and other leafy greens, may ease post-workout pain. Sulforaphane, a compound in these vegetables, seems to switch off a molecule that causes inflammation.

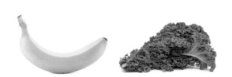

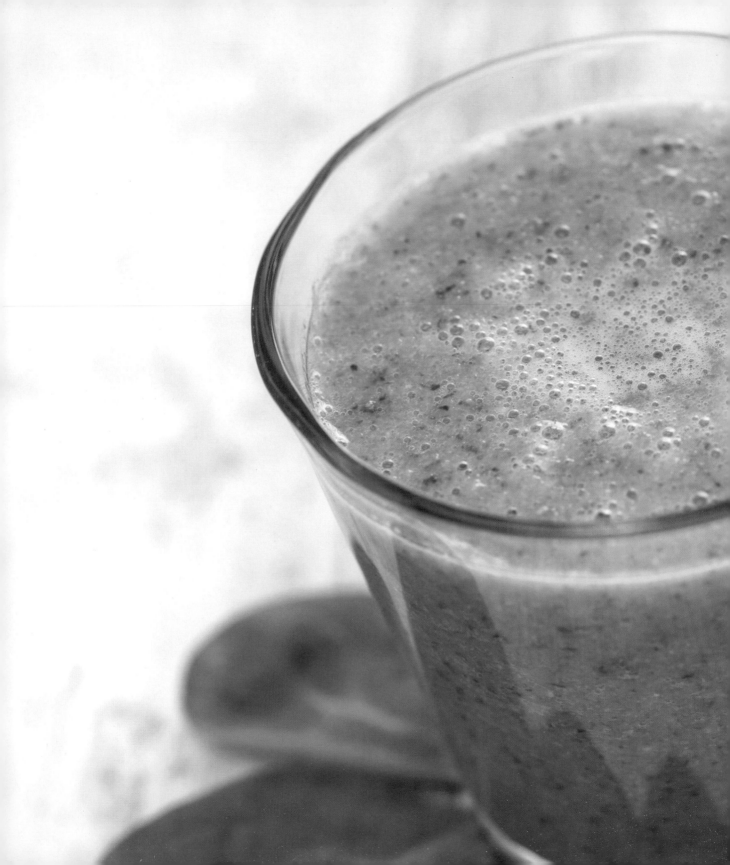

Green Goddess Smoothie {vegan friendly}

Looking for a breakfast that will fill you up and nourish you at the same time? This Green Goddess Smoothie will satisfy you all morning long while getting you closer to meeting daily nutrient requirements.

3 cups chopped spinach
½ apple
½ avocado, peeled and pitted
1 cup coconut water
4–5 ice cubes

Combine ingredients in a blender until smooth. Pour into a glass and serve immediately.

Spinach is one of the most nutrient-dense foods out there. It's loaded with vitamin K and vitamin A, manganese, and folate as well as fiber, calcium, and protein. It's also a good source of iron, which is essential to all-day energy.

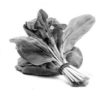

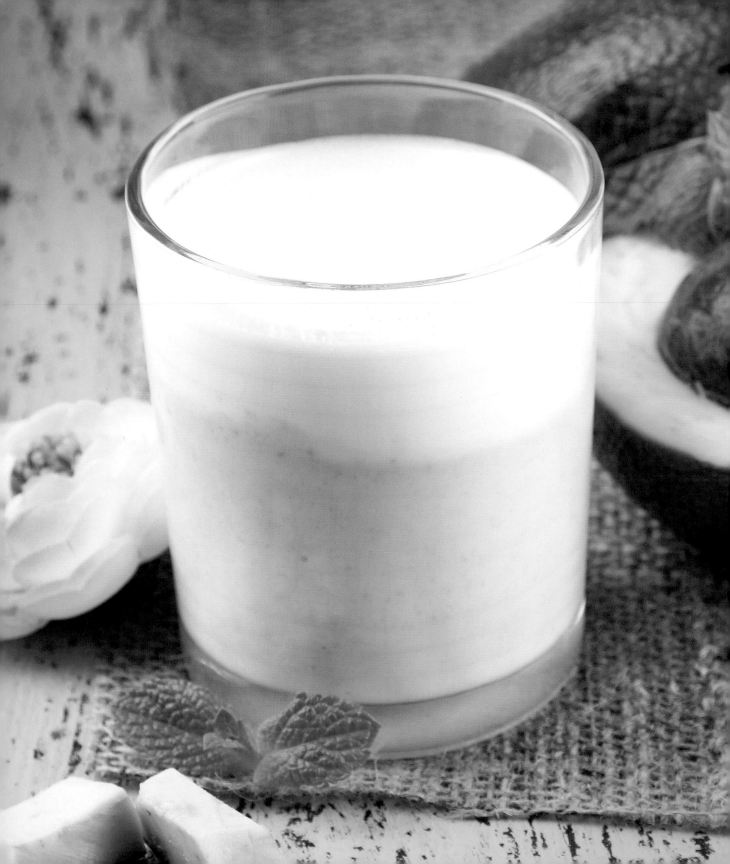

Minty Green Smoothie {vegan friendly}

As a natural pick-me-up, there's nothing better than fresh mint. It stimulates all of your senses! This smoothie takes it one step further by blending it with a bunch of especially tasty and nutritious ingredients.

3 cups chopped spinach (or kale)

½ pear

½ avocado, peeled and pitted

1 cup almond milk

10–12 leaves of fresh mint

4–5 ice cubes

Combine ingredients in a blender until smooth. Pour into a glass and serve immediately.

Mint is a natural stimulant, and the smell alone can be enough to boost your energy and help you focus.

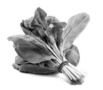

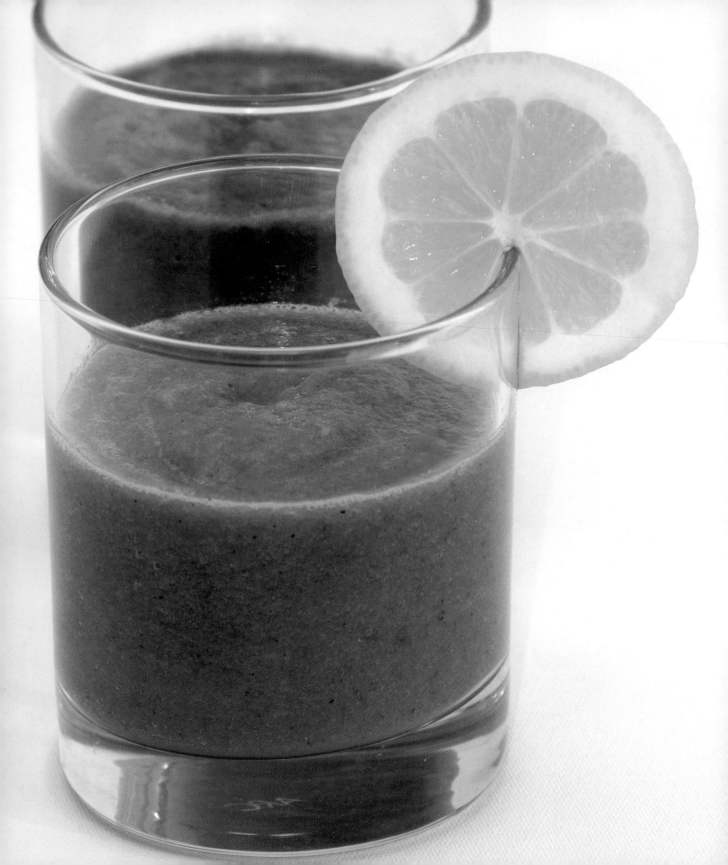

Green Lemonade Smoothie

Most lemonades are loaded with sugar, but this green version is instead packed with healthy nutrients.

1 large handful of spinach

1 lemon, peeled

½ banana

½ cucumber

½ cup water

2 tbsp honey (or agave nectar)

4–5 ice cubes

Combine ingredients in a blender until smooth. Pour into a glass and serve immediately.

> *"I believe that if life gives you lemons, you should make lemonade... And try to find somebody whose life has given them vodka, and have a party."*
>
> —RON WHITE

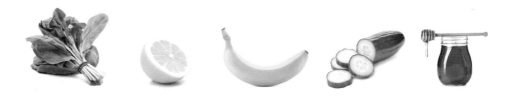

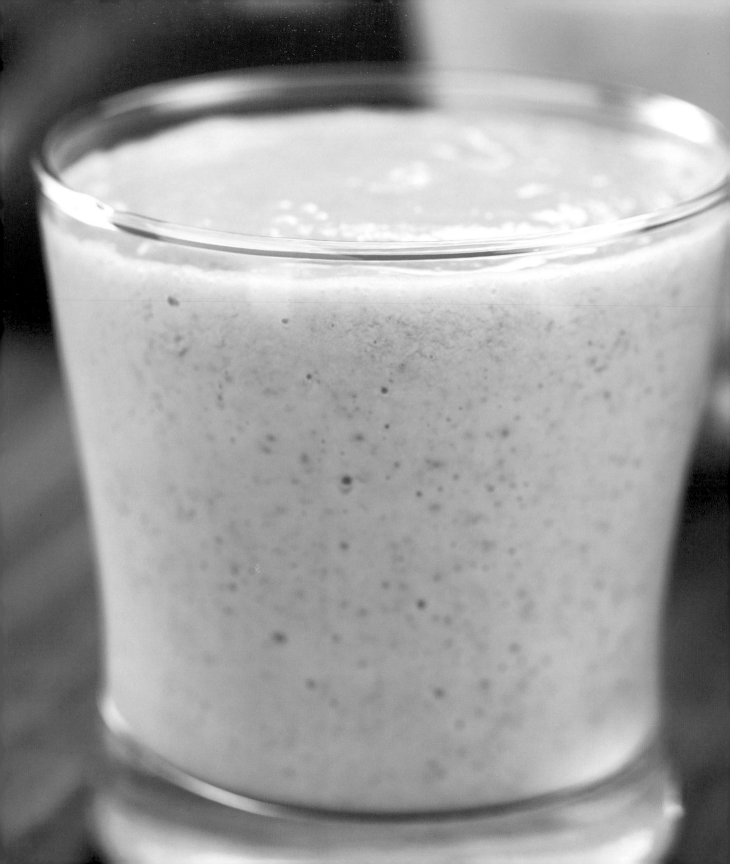

Emerald Island Smoothie

With this green smoothie, you'll enjoy a sweet taste of the tropics while getting a healthy dose of iron, vitamin C, and potassium thanks to the superstar cast of ingredients.

½ banana
½ cup frozen chunked pineapple
½ cup frozen chopped spinach
1 cup vanilla almond milk
1 tbsp honey (or agave nectar)

Combine ingredients in a blender until smooth. Pour into a glass and serve immediately.

Try this: Swap out the vanilla almond milk for chocolate almond milk.

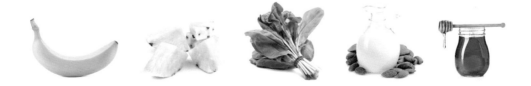

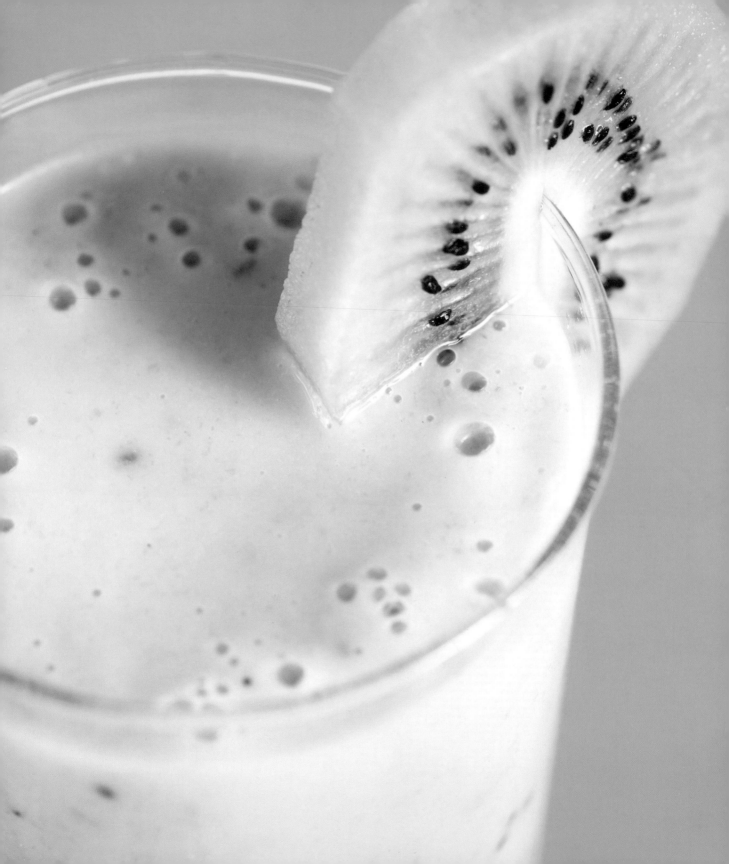

Mango Green Smoothie

Love mango? This smoothie is for you! You'll enjoy the delicious taste of mango mixed with sweet vanilla while getting your greens and protein for the day.

½ cup frozen mango chunks

½ cup frozen chopped spinach

1 kiwi, peeled

1.25 cups vanilla soy milk

1 scoop (25g) your choice of vanilla protein powder (optional)

Combine ingredients in a blender until smooth. Pour into a glass and serve immediately.

Try this: Omit spinach and add ½ cup of mixed frozen berries before blending.

 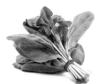

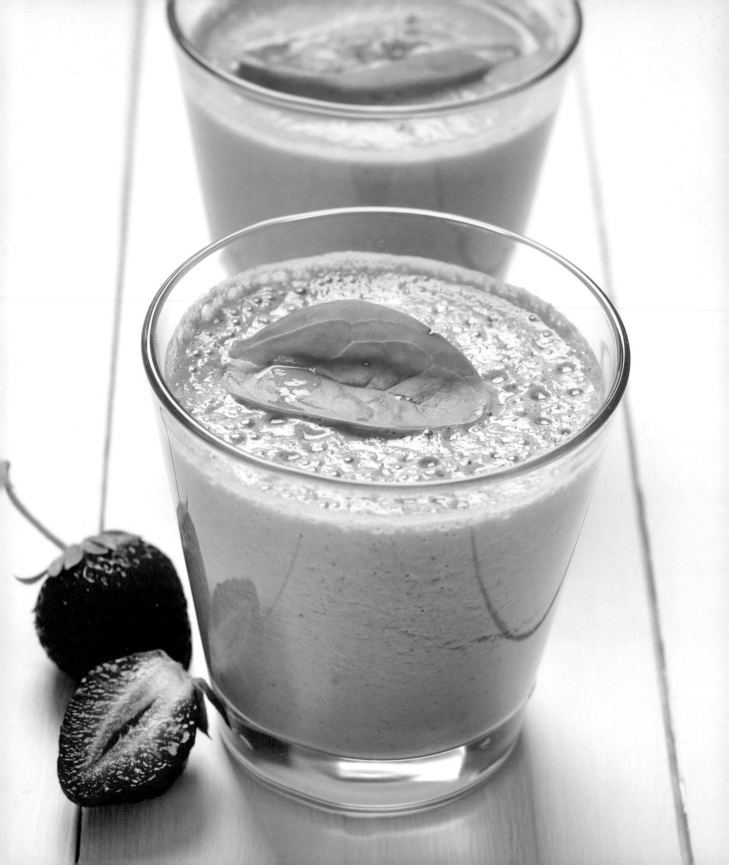

Sweet Green Smoothie {vegan friendly}

If you're not sure about the green smoothie trend, here's one that will ease you into it. Sweet strawberries, banana, and orange help mask the taste of spinach, so you'll get all of those important nutrients without even knowing it.

½ banana
½ cup frozen strawberries
1 large handful of spinach
½ cup orange (or apple) juice
½ cup vanilla almond milk
4–5 ice cubes

Combine ingredients in a blender until smooth. Pour into a glass and serve immediately.

> "It's bizarre that the produce manager is more important to my children's health than the pediatrician."
> —MERYL STREEP

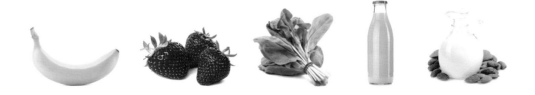

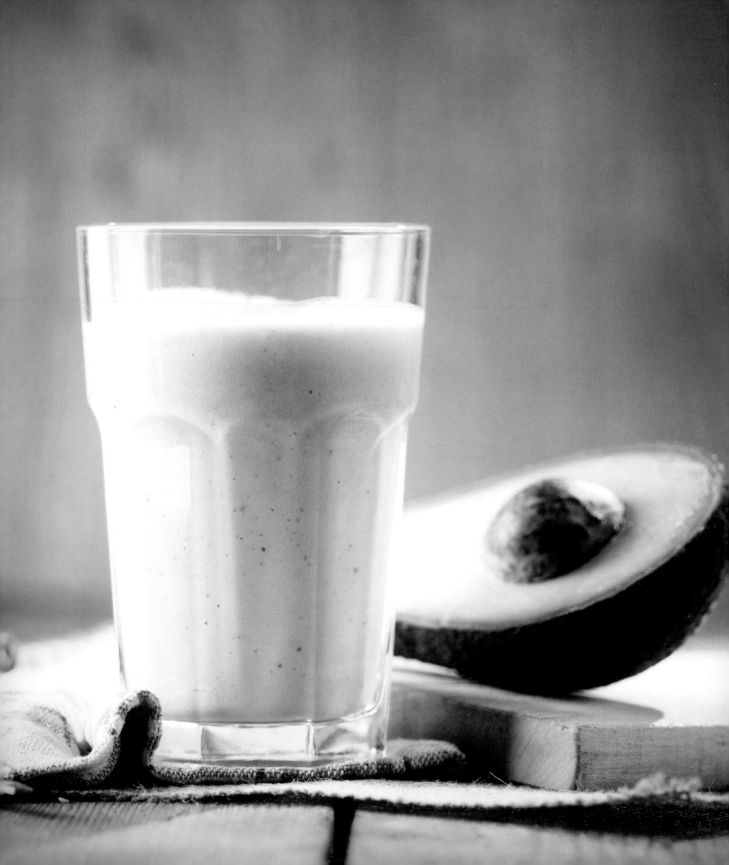

Creamy Avocado Smoothie

Avocado in a smoothie? You bet! It adds a wonderfully creamy texture and a colorful hue. This smoothie will seriously satisfy both your stomach and taste buds.

1 frozen banana
½ cup frozen chopped spinach
½ avocado, peeled and pitted
1.25 cups vanilla almond milk
1 tbsp honey (or agave nectar)
¼ tsp cinnamon

Combine ingredients in a blender until smooth. Pour into a glass and serve immediately.

Many people mistake avocado for a vegetable. But it's actually a fruit and, even more specifically, a single-seeded berry.

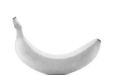 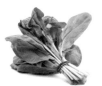

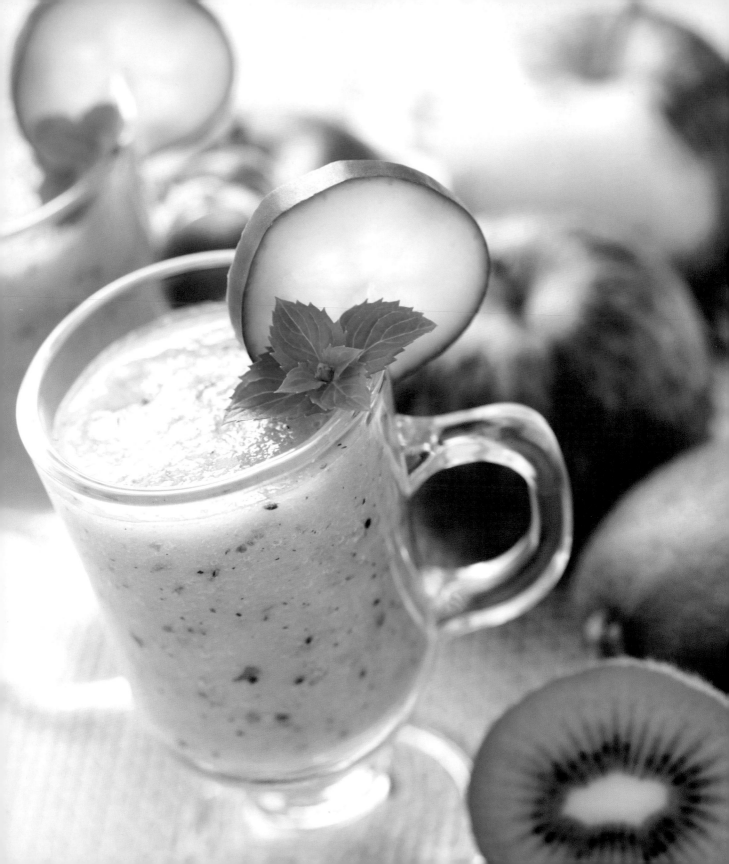

Apple-Cucumber-Kiwi Smoothie

Apple, cucumber, and kiwi combine in this light, refreshing smoothie. It's a little sweet, a little creamy, and a whole lot good for you.

1 apple, peeled, cored, and chopped

1 kiwi, peeled

½ cucumber, sliced

½ cup almond milk

2 tbsp almond butter

2 tsp honey (or agave nectar)

½ tsp cinnamon

4–5 ice cubes

Combine ingredients in a blender until smooth. Pour into a glass, garnish with a slice of cucumber if you'd like, and serve immediately.

Kiwi help to cleans out toxins in the body by binding and removing toxins from your intestinal tract.

  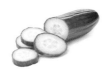

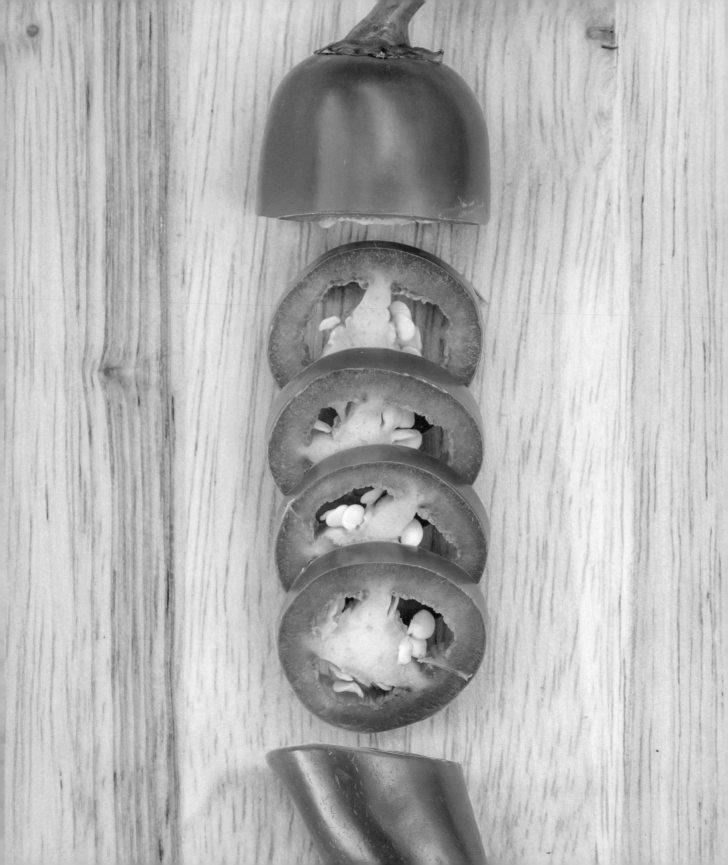

Spicy Green Smoothie {vegan friendly}

Ready for a little spice? This smoothie combines jalapeño and cayenne pepper for an exciting flavor. Drink this smoothie when you want a little zip in your life!

1 large handful of spinach

½ cucumber, cut into pieces

2 celery stalks

1 lemon, peeled

1 cup water

½ bunch of flat-leaf parsley

½ jalapeno, seeded

¼ tsp cayenne pepper

Pinch of sea salt

Combine ingredients in a blender until smooth. Pour into a glass and serve immediately.

A substance in jalapenos known as capsaicin may help boost your metabolism by raising the core temperature of the body— ultimately helping with weight loss. The metabolism-boosting effects of capsaicin are mild, but the hot flavor can help to lessen your appetite so you eat less at meals.

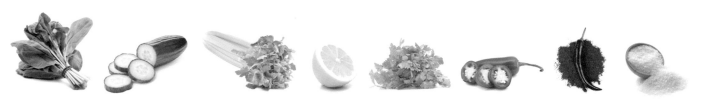

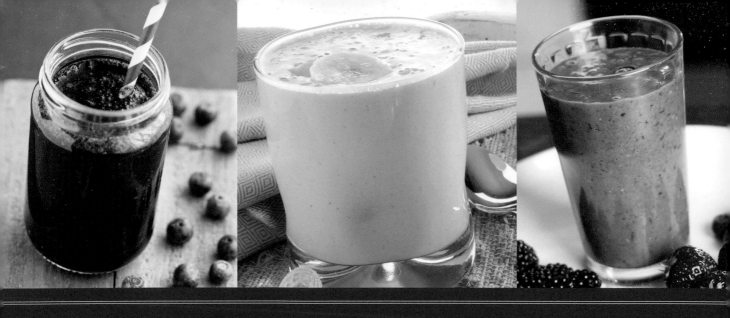

Chapter 4

Workout Smoothies

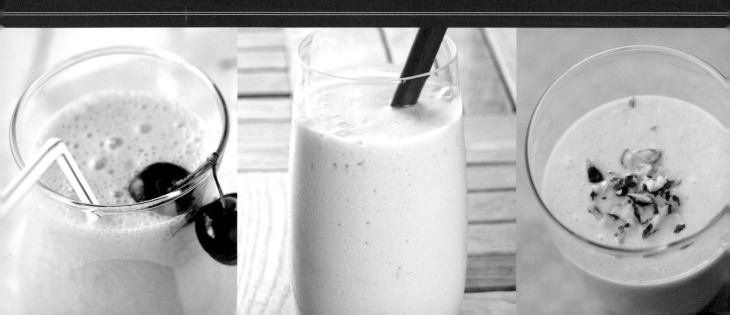

When it comes to fitness, if you've started to notice that your muscles don't recover as quickly as they used to and your performance is more sluggish than in the past, try focusing more on good post-workout nutrition. The key to proper recovery is consuming 10–20 grams of protein within 30 minutes of completing your workout. Drinking smoothies is a convenient way to get these essential nutrients in your diet.

The smoothies in this chapter include nutritious ingredients that help fight inflammation and promote quick repair and healing inside the body, which is especially important for overcoming soreness and getting you out the door for your next workout. All these recipes include nutritional powerhouse ingredients. From bananas and cherries to coconut water and chia seeds—you'll get the nutrients you need for recovery.

The majority of these smoothies call for protein powder, and there are lots of vegan varieties to choose from, including soy protein, pea protein, hemp protein, and rice protein. But, if you don't follow a strict plant-based diet, feel free to use the protein powder of your choice (e.g., whey, casein, egg white). Also, feel free to play around with the flavors of protein powder that you add to these smoothie recipes—a scoop of chocolate or coffee protein powder, for example, might just be the flavor you are looking for!

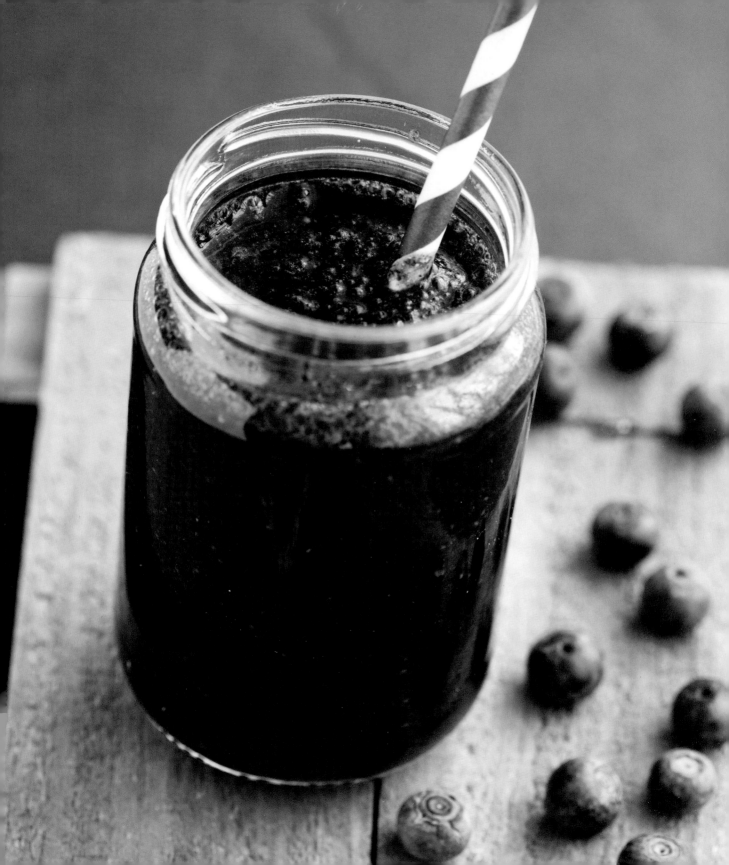

Ultimate Recovery Smoothie

This smoothie has an all-star cast of ingredients that are essential to proper recovery after a workout. For example, cherries have amazing anti-inflammatory powers and can help reduce post-workout soreness. This smoothie is delicious, too, making it one of my go-to options after a tough sweat session.

½ cup frozen cherries

½ cup frozen blueberries

½ cup chopped spinach

½ cup almond milk

½ cup coconut water

1 scoop (20g) your choice of **vanilla** protein powder

2 tsp chia seeds

Combine ingredients in a blender until smooth. Pour into a glass and enjoy immediately.

Try this: Swap out the frozen blueberries for ½ cup of frozen strawberries (or raspberries).

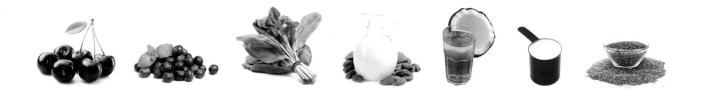

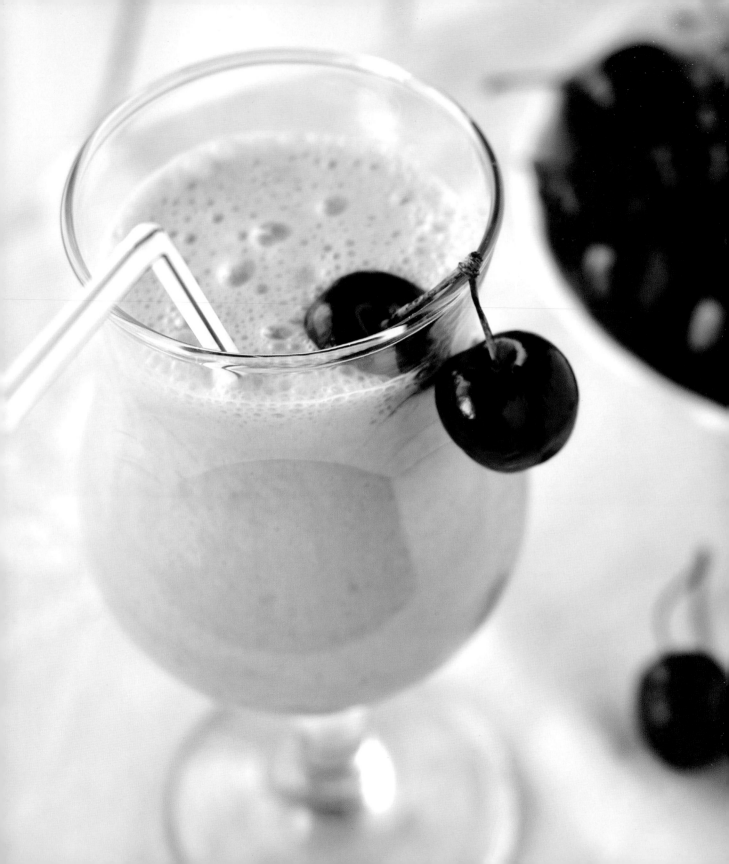

Cherry-Chocolate Smoothie

Made with cherries, banana, and honey (or agave nectar), this smoothie is a nutritional powerhouse. Studies show that combining honey with protein may boost post-workout recovery.

1 frozen banana
½ cup frozen cherries
1 cup chocolate soy milk
2 tsp honey (or agave nectar) (optional)
¼ tsp cinnamon

Combine ingredients in a blender until smooth. Pour into a glass and enjoy immediately.

Try this: For **more** chocolate taste, add 2 tablespoons of carob or dark chocolate chips **before** blending.

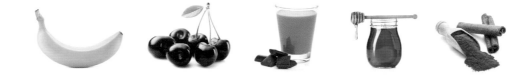

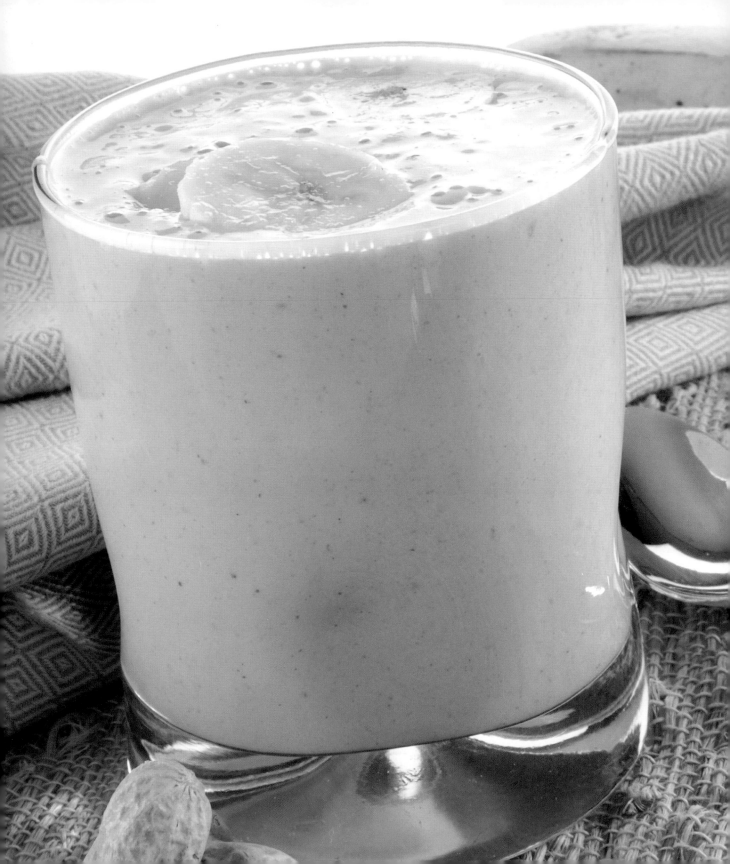

Best Peanut Butter and Banana Smoothie

Just about everyone has a favorite peanut butter and banana smoothie, but this one is truly the best. It's loaded with two heaping tablespoons of peanut butter to help you recover and keep you satisfied after your workout.

1 frozen banana

2 heaping tablespoons of peanut butter

1.25 cups vanilla almond milk

1 scoop (20g) your choice of vanilla protein powder

½ tsp vanilla extract

¼ tsp cinnamon

Combine ingredients in a blender until smooth. Pour into a glass and enjoy immediately.

Try this: Replace vanilla almond milk with chocolate almond milk.

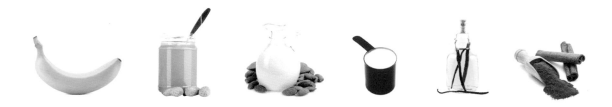

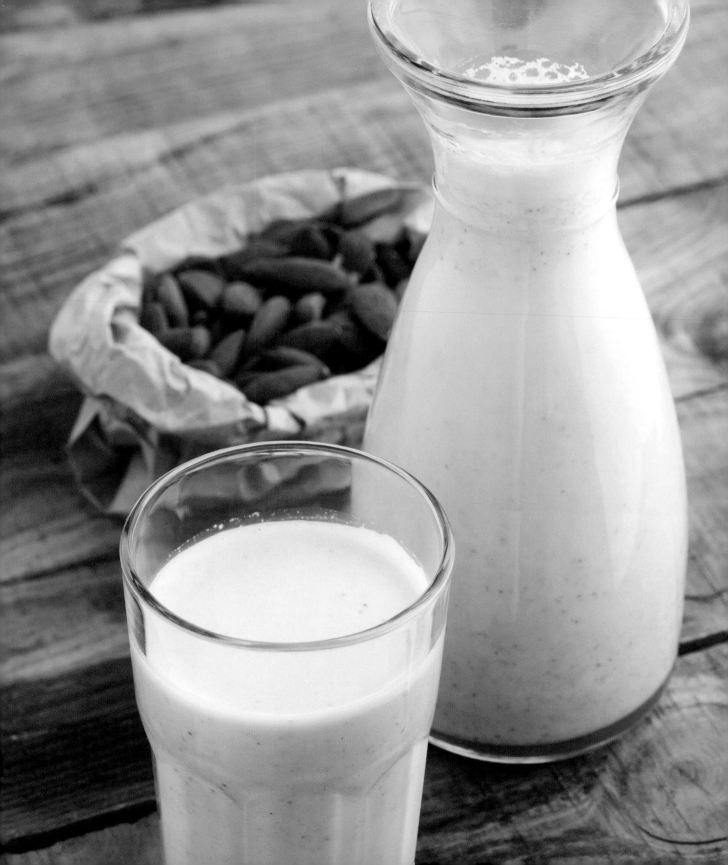

Vanilla Nut Smoothie

Sweet, nutty, and, oh, so delicious! Every time I make this smoothie, I slug it down in a matter of minutes, which is important for refueling muscles with essential vitamins and minerals immediately after exercise.

1 frozen banana

2 tbsp almond butter

1.25 cup vanilla almond milk

1 scoop (20g) your choice of vanilla protein powder

1 tbsp ground flaxseed meal

1 tbsp maple syrup

Combine ingredients in a blender until smooth. Pour into a glass and enjoy immediately.

Nuts, like almonds, are beneficial for maintaining a healthy weight. The fiber, protein, and fat content of almonds helps to keep you feeling full and satisfied so you won't have the urge to overeat later on.

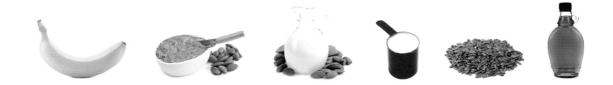

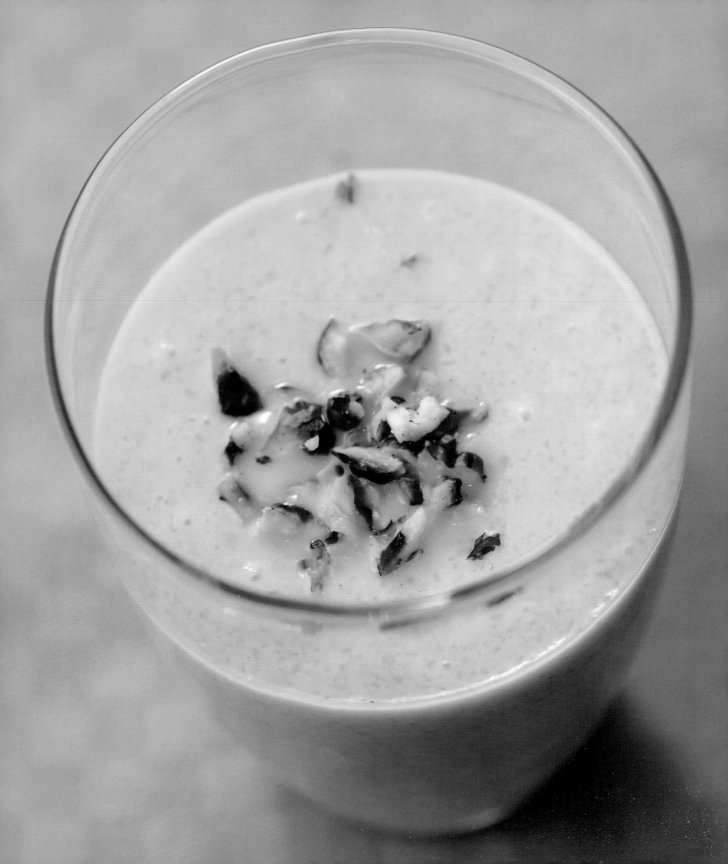

Sweet Potato Pie Protein Smoothie

This superfood smoothie sure tastes delicious, and the combination of protein and complex carbohydrates will also help refuel and repair tired muscles after a tough workout.

½ cup mashed sweet potato

½ frozen banana

¾ cup vanilla soy milk

1 scoop (20g) your choice of **vanilla** protein powder

1 tbsp maple syrup

½ tsp cinnamon

Dash of nutmeg (optional)

4–5 ice cubes

Combine ingredients in a blender until smooth. Pour into a glass and enjoy immediately.

Sweet potatoes provide a healthy dose of complex carbohydrates for sustained energy, so eat them before your workouts, too!

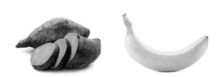

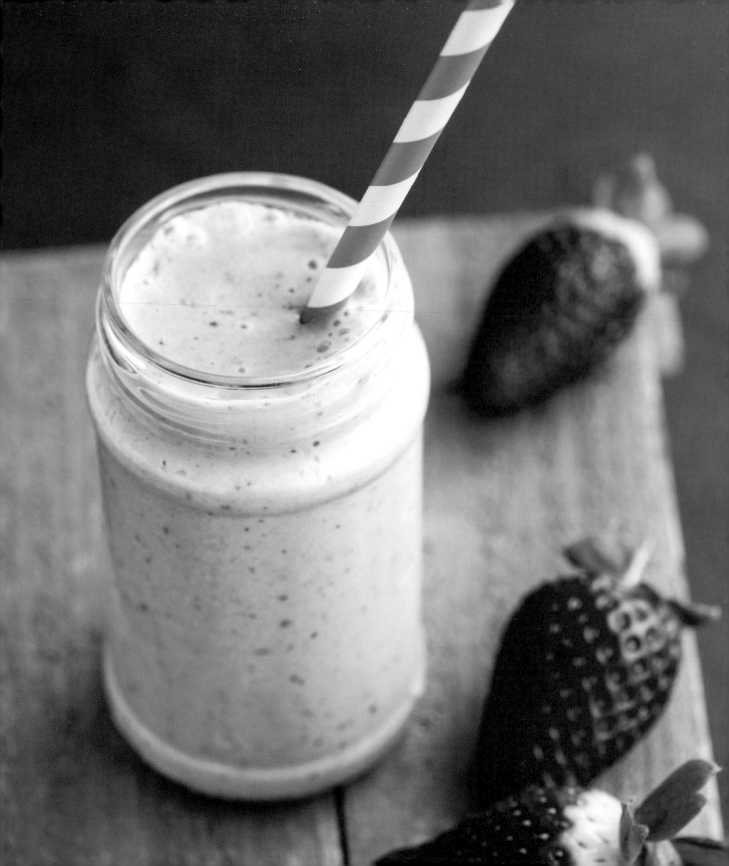

Strawberry-Almond Smoothie

Strawberries and almonds come together in this dessert-like smoothie. You might think the taste is too good to be true, but it's actually a wonderful recovery smoothie too, thanks to all of the muscle-repairing nutrients.

1 cup frozen strawberries

2 tbsp almond butter

1.5 cup vanilla almond milk

1 scoop (20g) your choice of **vanilla** protein powder

2 tbsp sliced almonds (optional)

Combine ingredients in a blender until smooth. Pour into a glass and enjoy immediately.

For optional post-workout recovery, consume 10–20 grams of protein within 30 minutes of completing your workout.

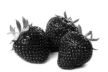 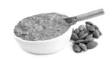

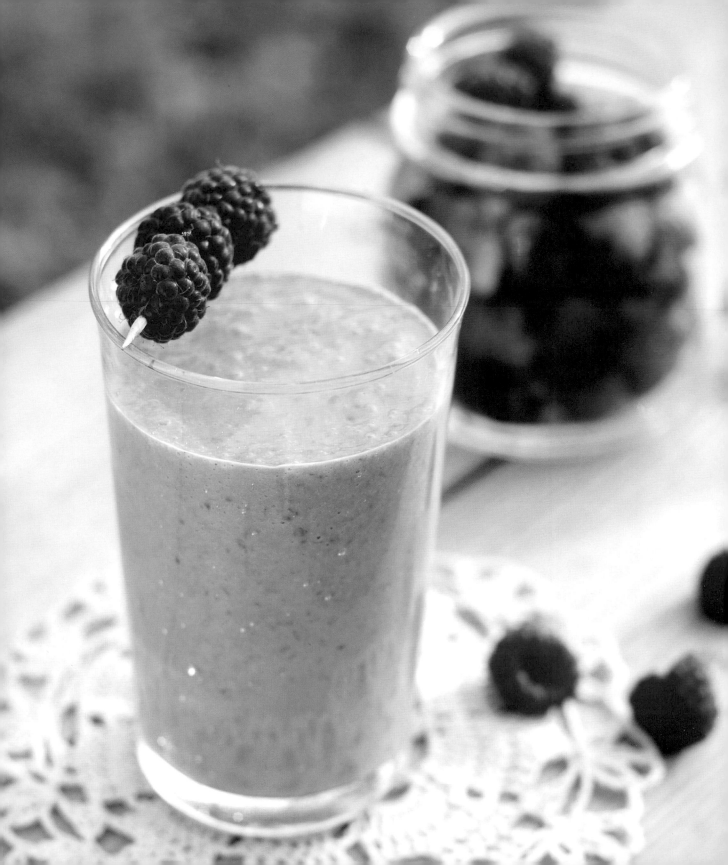

Coco-Choco-Raspberry Smoothie

Rehydrate and replenish with this delicious smoothie made with raspberries, spinach, coconut, and protein powder.

1 cup frozen raspberries

2 cups baby spinach

1 cup coconut milk

¼ cup coconut water

1 scoop (20g) chocolate-flavored protein powder

2 tbsp shredded coconut

Combine ingredients in a blender until smooth. Pour into a glass and enjoy immediately.

Coconut water is rich in electrolytes and potassium, which makes it great for rehydration after exercise.

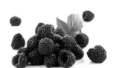 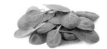

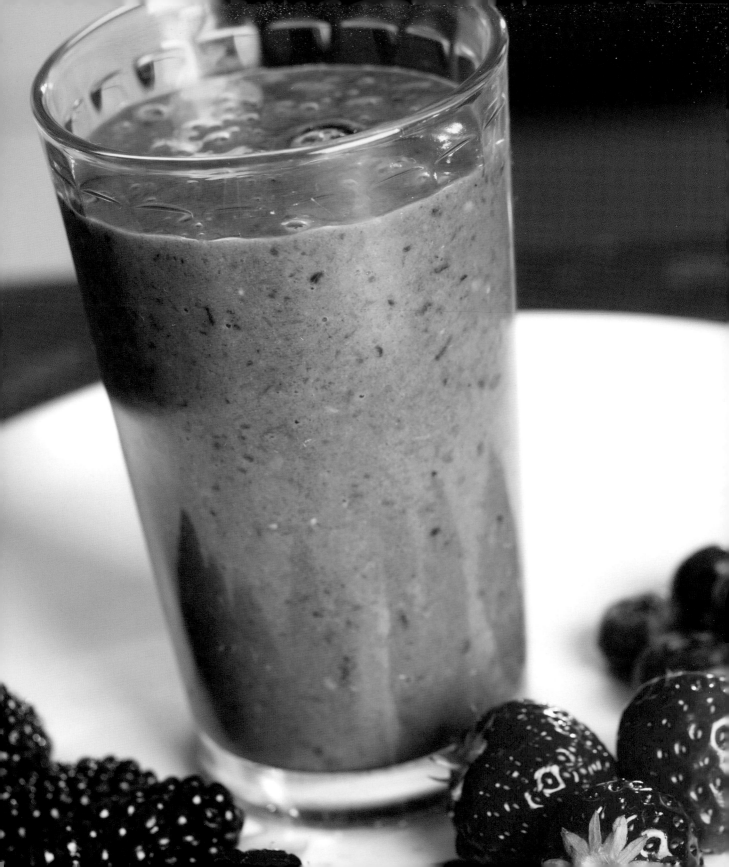

Pineapple-Berry Protein Smoothie

This smoothie is loaded with good-for-you antioxidants and bromelain (from the pineapple) to help fight inflammation and help your body recover more quickly after a workout.

½ cup frozen pineapple chunks

½ cup frozen mixed berries

1.25 cups almond milk

1 scoop (20g) your choice of vanilla protein powder

Combine ingredients in a blender until smooth. Pour into a glass and enjoy immediately.

Pineapple contains bromelain, an enzyme that helps reduce inflammation in the body. It's also a good source of vitamin C, which helps strengthen your immune system.

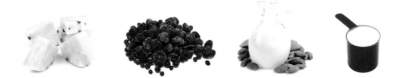

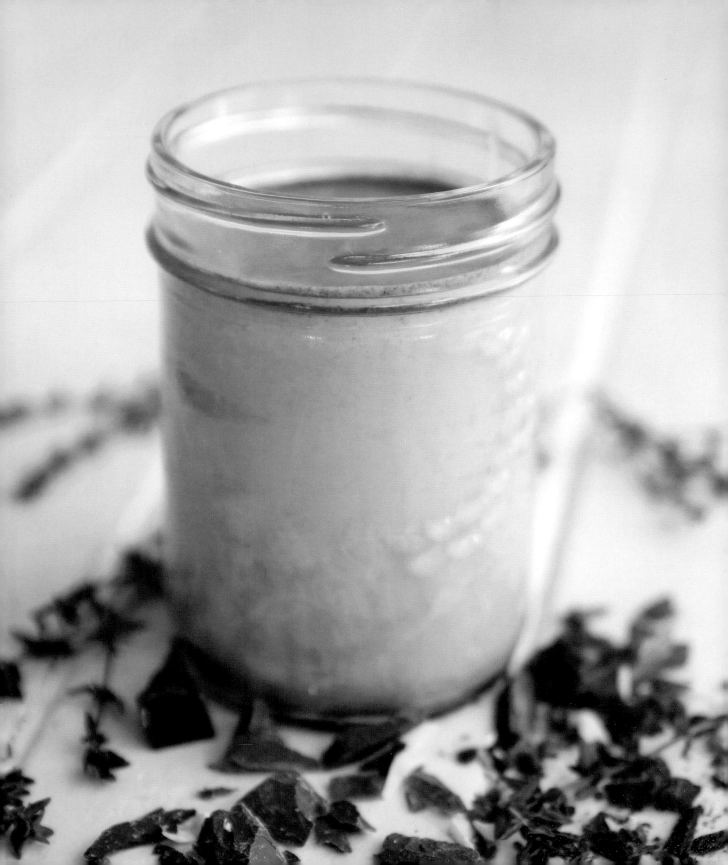

Creamy Chocolate Protein Smoothie

Tough workout? If so, you might be looking for a sweet reward for all of your hard work. This smoothie provides protein to your muscles for quick recovery while tasting like a delectable chocolate dessert at the same time!

1 frozen banana

½ cup frozen chopped spinach

½ avocado, peeled and pitted

1.25 cups chocolate almond milk

1 scoop (25g) your choice of chocolate protein powder

2 tsp chia seeds (optional)

Combine ingredients in a blender until smooth. Pour into a glass and enjoy immediately.

Chia seeds can enhance your training and improve your overall healthy in a number of ways, from combating dehydration and reducing inflammation to promoting weight loss and accelerating post-workout recovery.

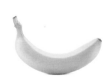 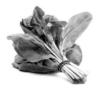

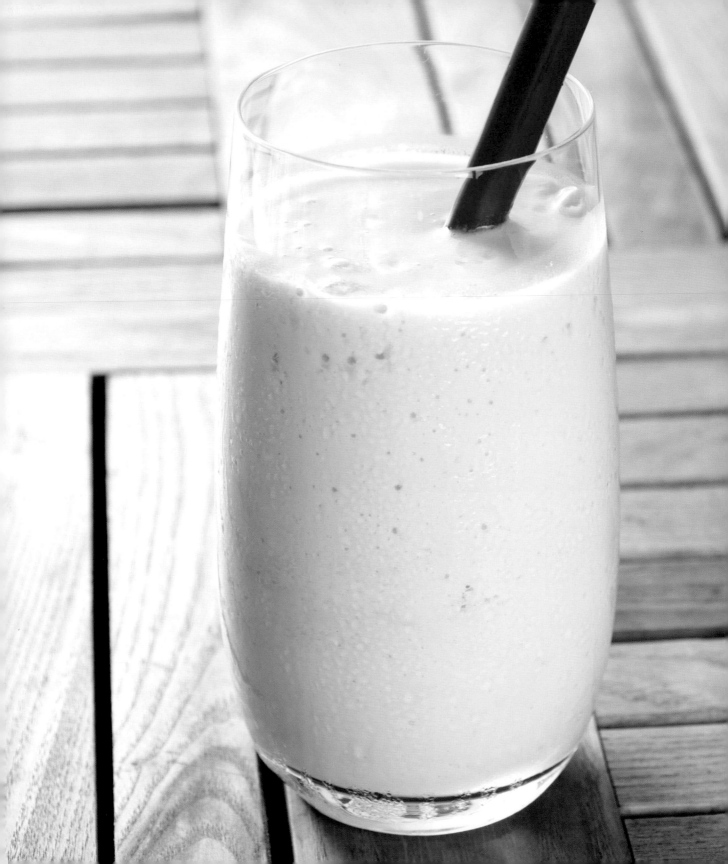

Squash Soreness Smoothie

The variety of nutrients in this smoothie promote quick repair and healing after a workout, which is important for overcoming soreness and getting you out the door for your next sweat session.

½ banana

½ cup frozen pineapple chunks

½ cup frozen diced butternut squash

1 scoop (20g) your choice of vanilla protein powder

1 cup coconut water

2 tsp honey (or agave nectar)

1 tsp chia seeds

¼ tsp cinnamon

Combine ingredients in a blender until smooth. Pour into a glass and enjoy immediately.

Try this: Replace coconut water with 1 cup of pomegranate juice.

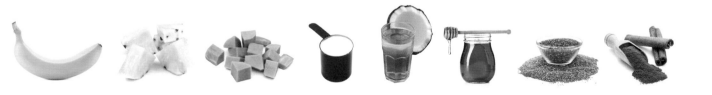

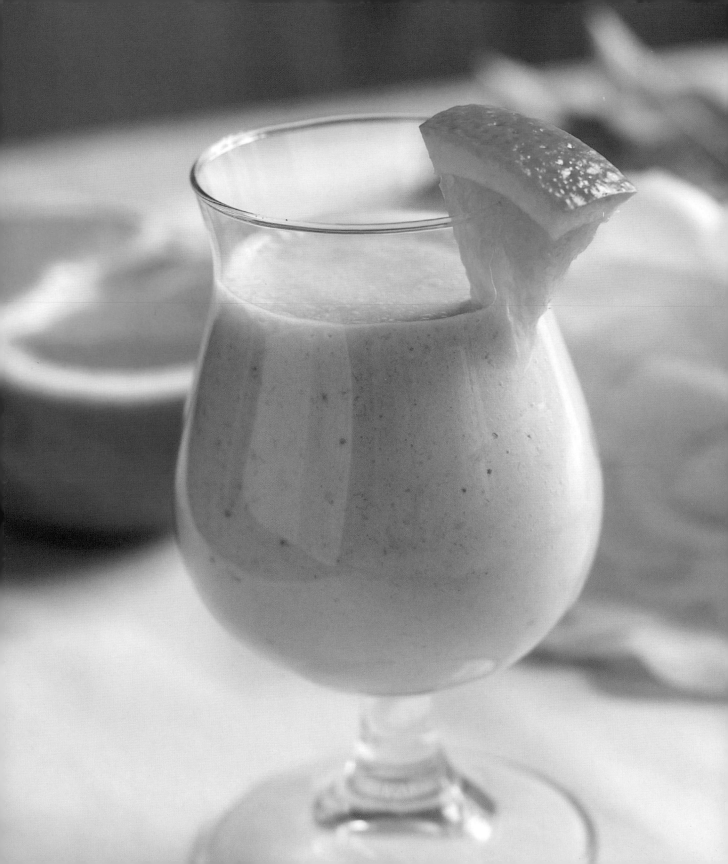

Orange Creamsicle Smoothie

You finished a tough workout! Congrats! How about a cool, sweet, and creamy treat to reward yourself? This Orange Creamsicle Smoothie will make all of your hard work worth it without adding a ton of calories to your diet.

1 cup orange juice

6–8 ounces vanilla-flavored yogurt

½ frozen banana

1 scoop (20g) your choice of vanilla protein powder

2 tsp honey (or agave nectar) (optional)

4–5 ice cubes

Combine ingredients in a blender until smooth. Pour into a glass and enjoy immediately.

A single cup of orange juice can meet more than 100 percent of your daily requirement of Vitamin C. This vital nutrient helps improve your immunity, which helps prevents diseases and infections.

  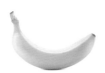

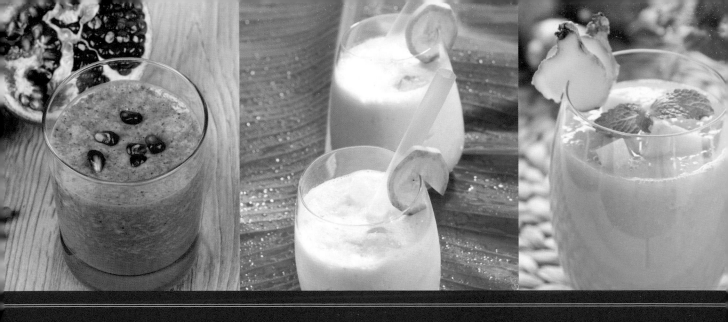

Chapter 5

Energizing Smoothies

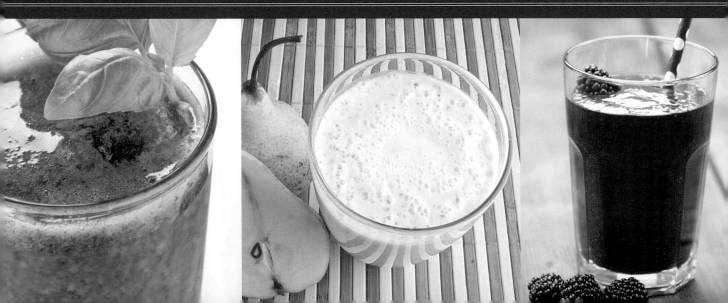

*I*f you struggle with getting moving in the morning or tend to feel a bit sluggish in the afternoon, an energizing smoothie, packed full of nutrients and feel-good ingredients, is exactly just what you need!

These recipes include a variety of ingredients that will give you a natural boost: tropical fruits, refreshing mint, zippy fresh ginger, and iron-rich leafy greens. Whip up one of these smoothies any time you need a lift.

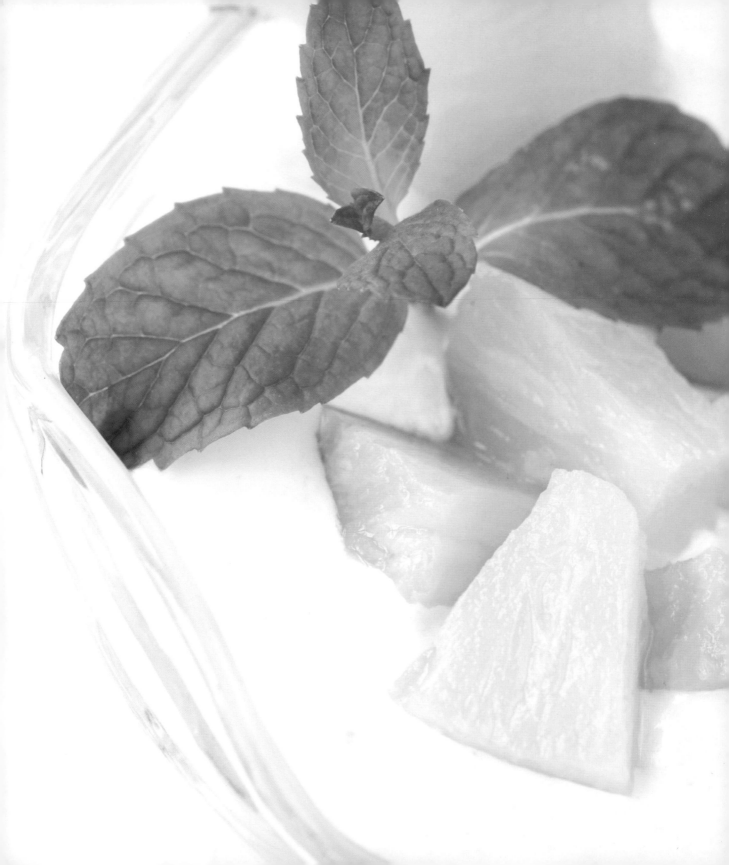

Tropical Mint Smoothie

Sweet, creamy, and refreshing, this tropical-tasting smoothie is the perfect pick-me-up!

1 frozen banana
½ cup crushed pineapple (fresh or canned)
1 cup coconut milk
1 tsp honey (or agave nectar)
8–10 fresh mint leaves

Combine ingredients in a blender until smooth. Pour into a glass and enjoy immediately.

Try this: Replace the crushed pineapple with ½ cup of cubed mango.

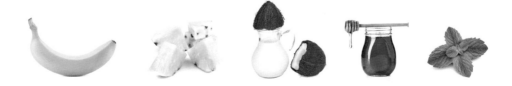

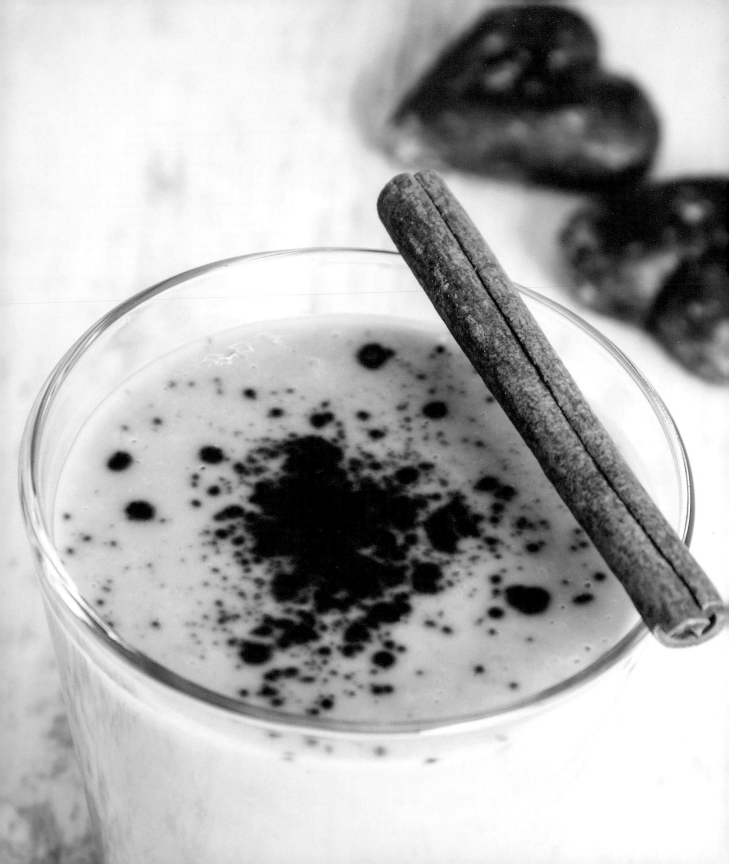

Java Jolt Smoothie

Need a little pick-me-up? Look no further! This smoothie will give you the energy you need to help you sail through your day.

1 frozen banana
2 tbsp almond butter
1 cup almond milk
1 ounce espresso
1 tsp honey (or agave nectar)
½ tsp vanilla extract
½ tsp cinnamon
4–5 ice cubes

Combine ingredients in a blender until smooth. Pour into a glass, garnish with a cinnamon stick if desired, and enjoy immediately.

Try this: Add 2 tablespoons of carob or dark chocolate chips.

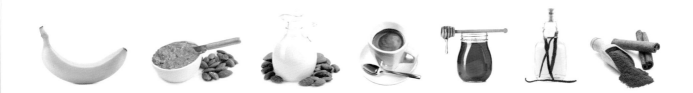

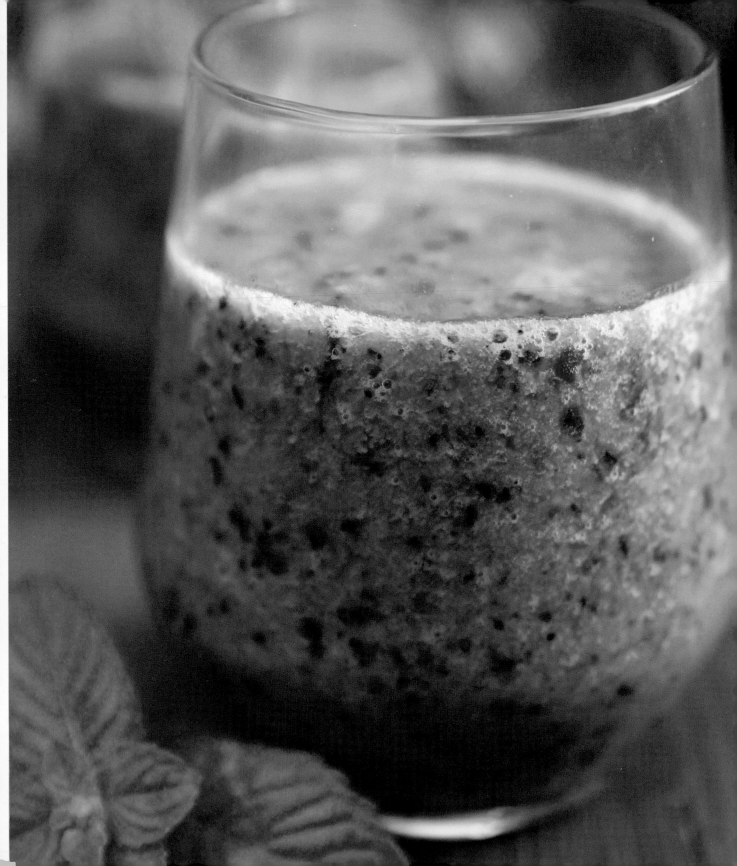

Mint-Berry Smoothie

This creamy berry smoothie with fresh mint will really wow you! You're sure to love the fresh and fruity flavor combination of the berries, banana, apple, honey (or agave nectar), and mint.

½ banana
½ cup frozen mixed berries
1 apple, cored and chopped
½ cup water
2 tsp honey (or agave nectar) (optional)
10–12 fresh mint leaves

Combine ingredients in a blender until smooth. Pour into a glass and enjoy immediately.

Mint contains a phytonutrient called *perillyl alcohol* that may play a role in halting tumors and preventing cancer of the lungs, colon, and skin.

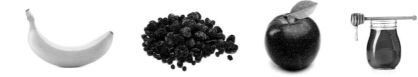

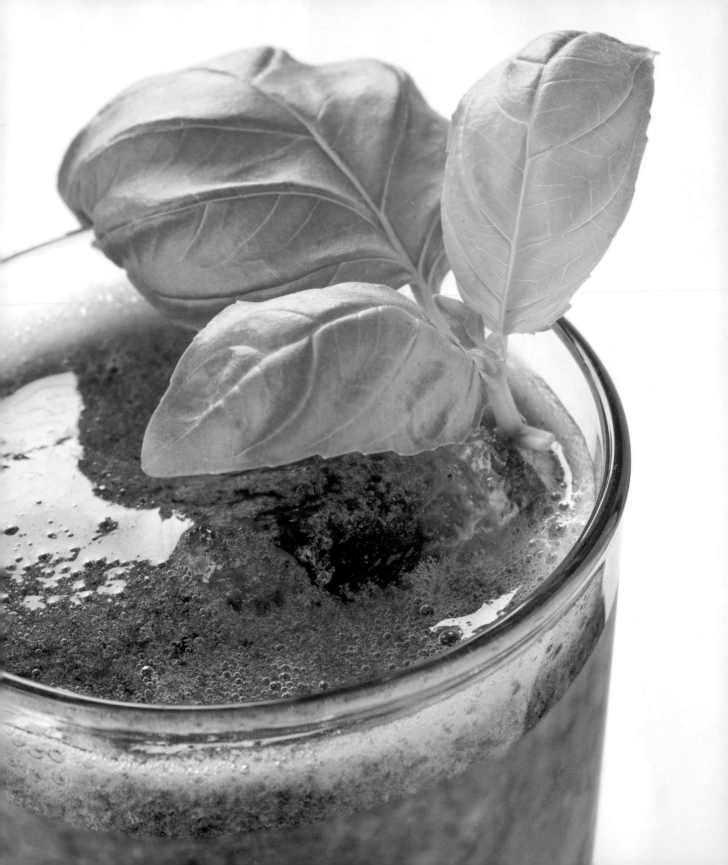

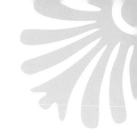

Strawberry-Basil Smoothie {vegan friendly}

You can enjoy this summery flavor combination all year long with this Strawberry-Basil Smoothie.

¾ cup strawberries

½ frozen banana

1.25 cup almond milk

1 tbsp freshly squeezed lemon juice (optional)

A small handful of fresh basil leaves (approximately 10–12)

Combine ingredients in a blender until smooth. Pour into a glass, garnish with fresh basil if you'd like, and enjoy immediately.

Try this: For a Strawberry-Basil Lemonade Smoothie, omit almond milk and add a peeled lemon and 4–5 ice cubes before blending.

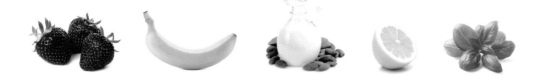

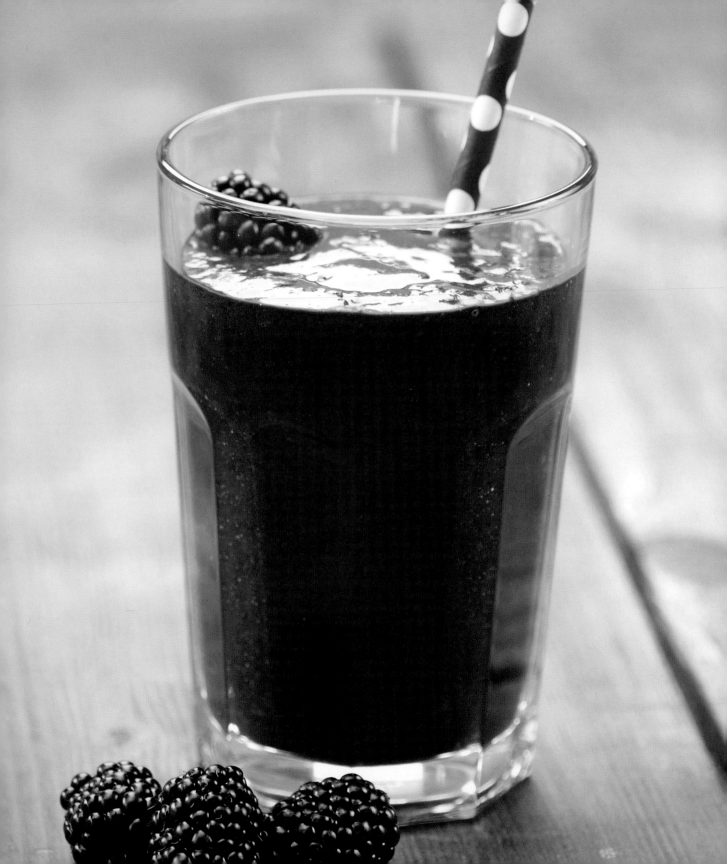

Blackberry-Coconut Smoothie

Both sweet and tart, the taste of blackberries mixed with coconut will practically melt in your mouth. You'll want to enjoy this soft, succulent flavor again and again.

1 frozen banana

¾ cup frozen blackberries

1.5 cups coconut milk

1 tbsp honey (or agave nectar)

¼ tsp coconut extract

1 tbsp shredded coconut (optional)

Combine ingredients in a blender until smooth. Pour into a glass and enjoy immediately.

What's a blackberry by another name? Brambleberries, dewberries, or thimbleberries.

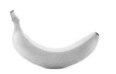

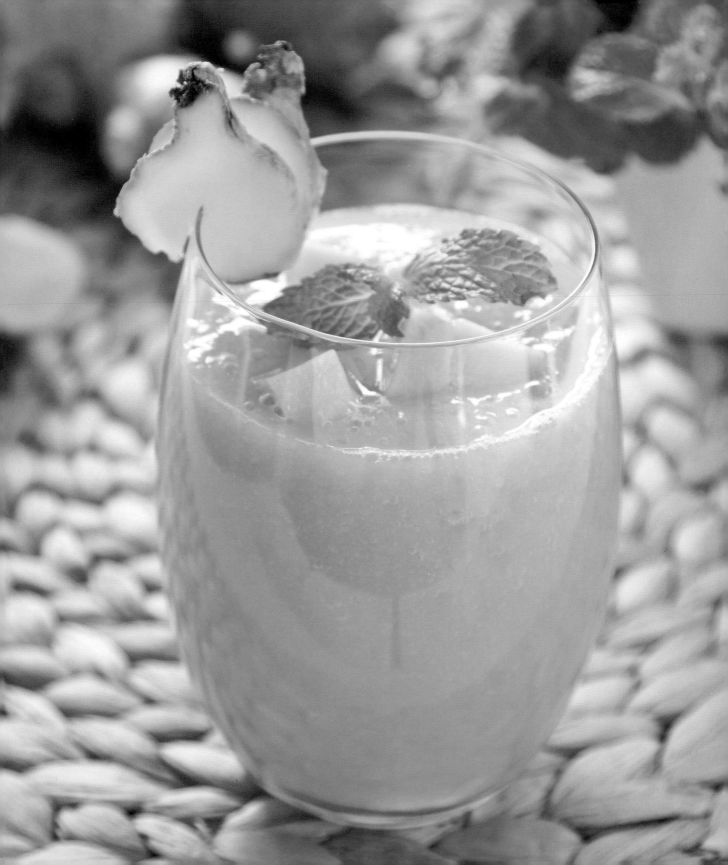

Pineapple Zinger Smoothie {vegan friendly}

Citrus and ginger are a winning combination in this smoothie. From the first sip, you'll feel more awake and energized. The iron in the spinach also gives your body a little boost.

1 cup frozen chunked pineapple

⅓ cup frozen chopped spinach

¾ cup orange juice

¾ cup almond milk

1 tbsp freshly grated ginger

Combine ingredients in a blender until smooth. Pour into a glass, garnish with sliced ginger if desired, and enjoy immediately.

It takes about 20 months for a pineapple plant to produce a single fruit and another 14–15 months to produce a second fruit.

 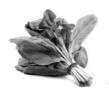

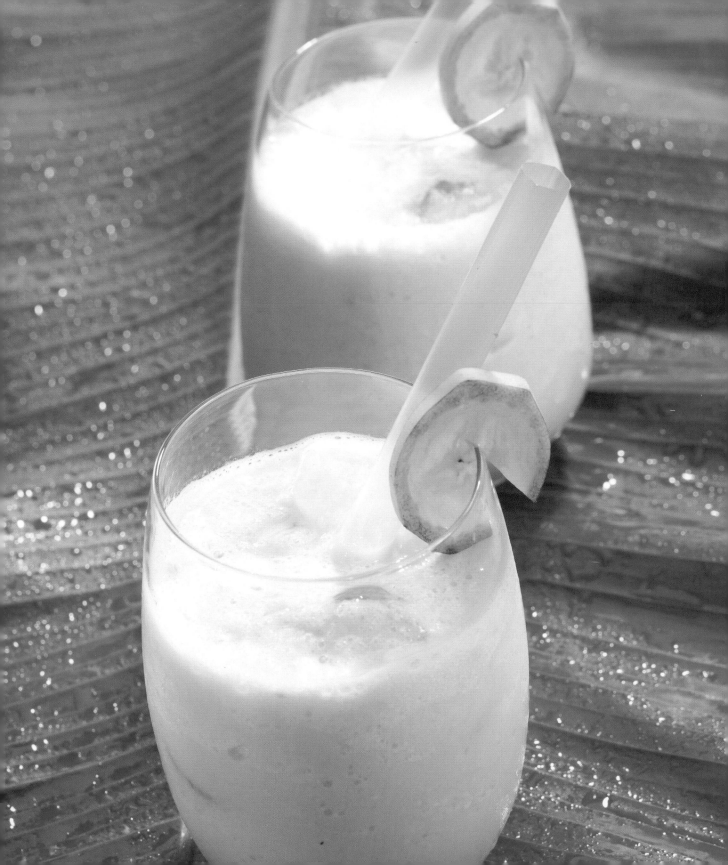

Island Time Smoothie

Sit back and relax with this tropical-inspired smoothie. The flavors of pineapple, mango, and coconut will sweep you away. You're on island time now!

½ cup of chunked pineapple
½ cup chunked mango
1.75 cup of vanilla almond milk
2 tbsp shredded coconut
¼ tsp coconut extract
2 tsp honey (optional)

Combine ingredients in a blender until smooth. Pour into a glass and enjoy immediately. Sunglasses optional.

> *"The sun and the sand and a drink in my hand..."*
> —KENNY CHESNEY

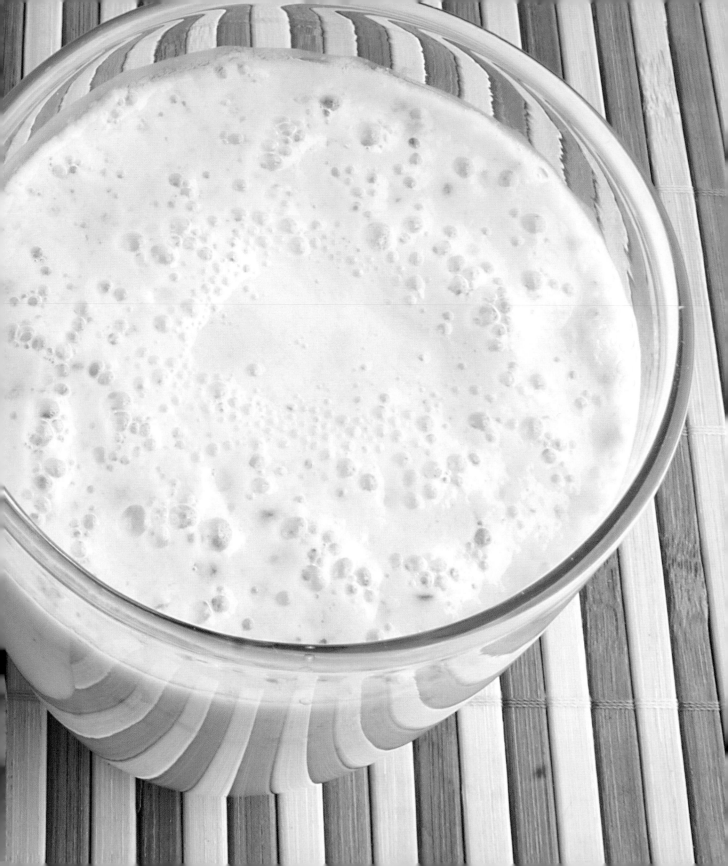

Gingerbread Smoothie

Craving something sweet this afternoon? Here's the smoothie for you!
It tastes like you're enjoying a cool, creamy gingerbread cookie but for
a fraction of the calories and many more vitamins and nutrients.

1 pear, diced

1 cup almond milk

1 scoop of your choice of vanilla
protein powder

½ tsp cinnamon

¼ tsp ground ginger

4–5 ice cubes

Combine ingredients in a blender until smooth.
Pour into a glass and enjoy immediately.

Traditionally, gingerbread was
used to treat indigestion and
upset stomachs.

 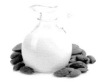

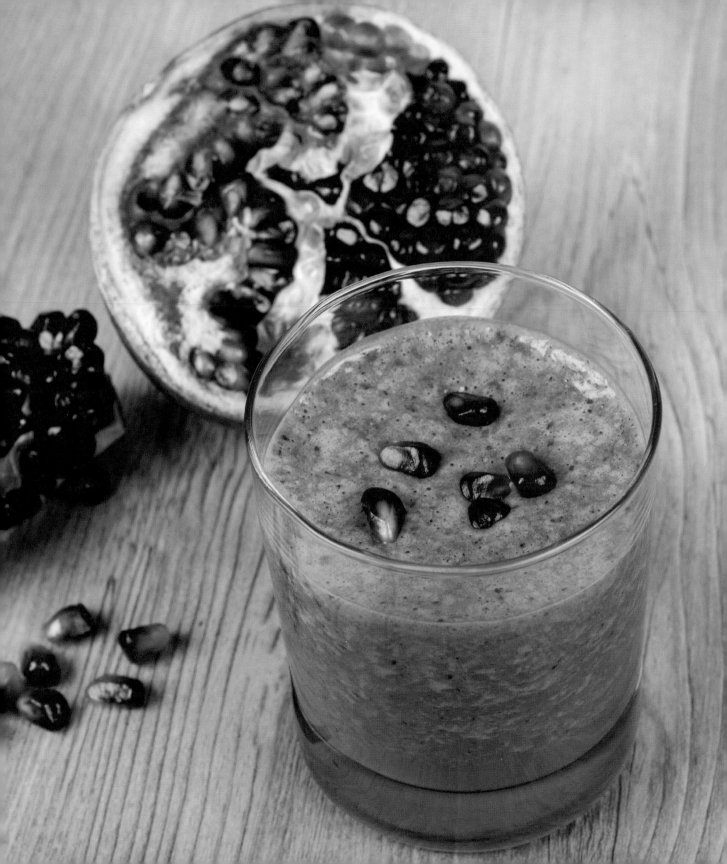

Pineapple-Pomegranate Smoothie {vegan friendly}

Made with satisfying avocado and taste bud–tantalizing pineapple and pomegranate juice, this smoothie will ward off hunger and give you a natural pick-me-up.

1 cup chunked frozen pineapple
½ avocado, peeled and pitted
¾ cup pomegranate juice
½ cup almond milk

Combine ingredients in a blender until smooth. Pour into a glass and enjoy immediately.

Try this: Replace pineapple with 1 cup of frozen mango.

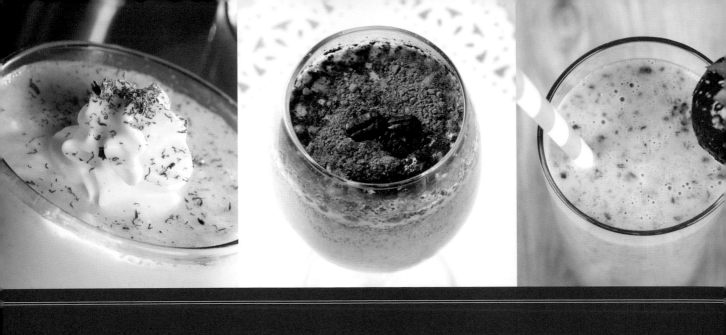

Chapter 6

Dessert Smoothies

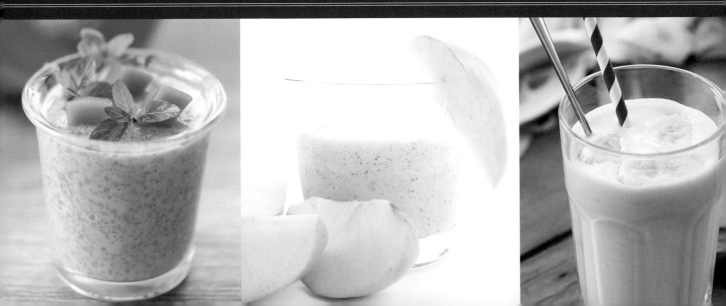

*W*e all love dessert, right? But, of course, these decadent treats are not typically low in calories or friendly on the waistline. Instead of missing out on the fun and great taste of your favorite sweet treats, try dessert smoothies. You'll enjoy the best of both worlds: a decadent dessert loaded with good-for-you-ingredients. It really doesn't get better than that!

You'll recognize the flavors in this chapter as some of your favorite desserts, including Peanut Butter Cup, Oatmeal Raisin Cookie, and Bananas Foster. Lucky for us, these delicious dessert blends are just a fraction of the calories and fat of the traditional versions, which means you can enjoy them without guilt.

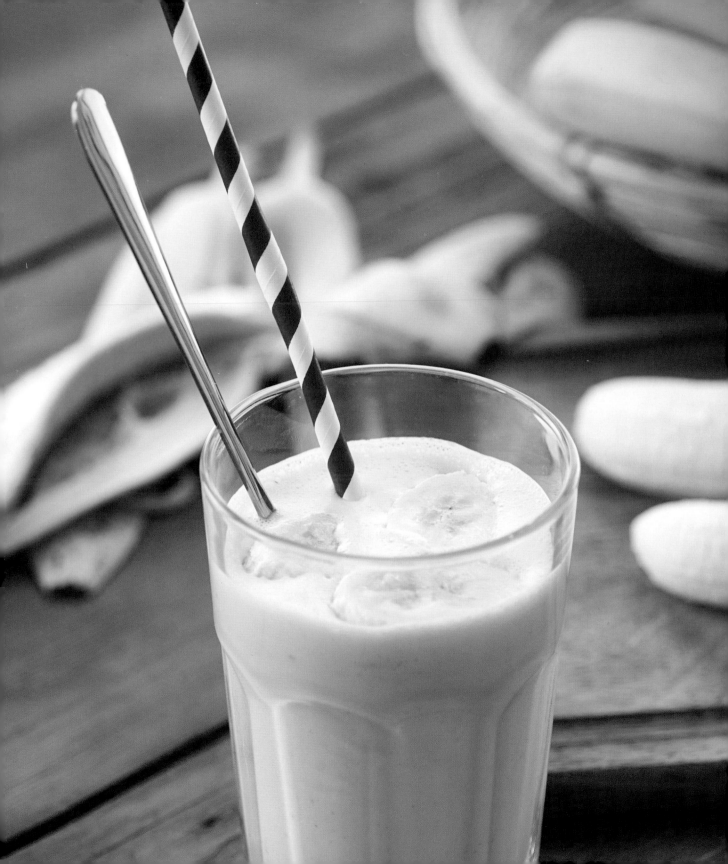

Banana Foster Smoothie {vegan friendly}

Banana Foster is a decadent classic dessert, but it's not low in calories or friendly on the waistline. Try this lighter, smoothie version! You may even like it better.

1 frozen banana

1 cup vanilla almond milk

6–8 pecans

2 tsp brown sugar

½ tsp rum extract

¼ tsp vanilla extract

Combine ingredients in a blender until smooth. Pour into a glass and enjoy immediately.

Try this: For a **coffee**-flavored dessert-like smoothie, add 1 ounce of espresso or strongly **brewed** coffee.

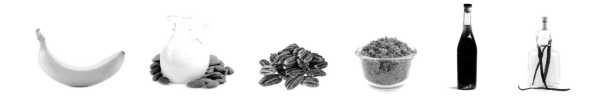

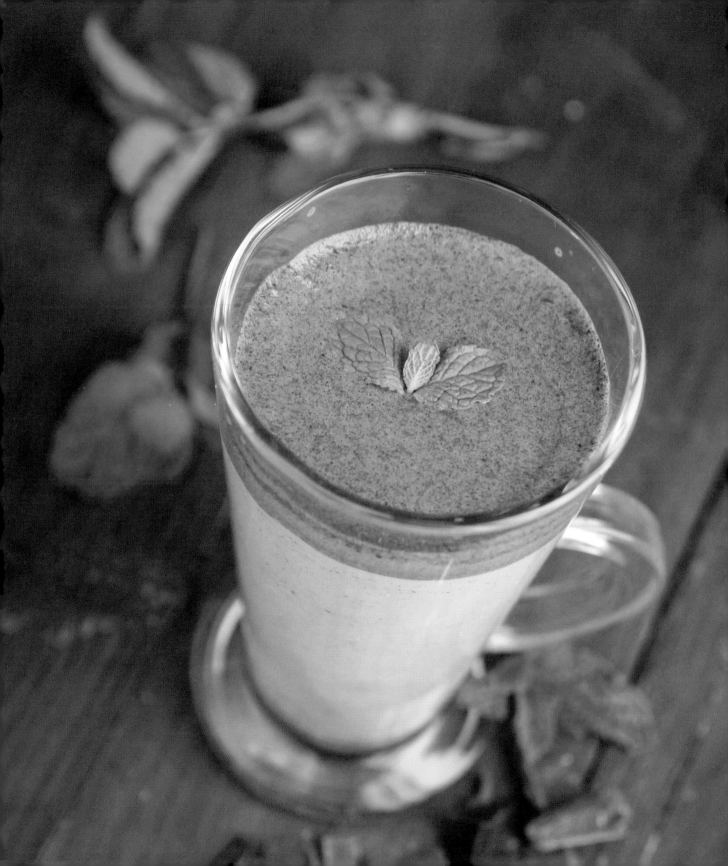

Thin Mint Smoothie

Mint and chocolate together? The pairing is an instant flavor favorite. This smoothie uses fresh mint for a seriously intense yet playful flavor punch.

1 frozen banana

1.25 cups vanilla almond milk

2 tbsp carob or dark chocolate chips

8–10 leaves of fresh mint

¼ tsp peppermint extract (optional)

Combine ingredients in a blender until smooth. Pour into a glass, garnish with a fresh mint leaf if you'd like, and enjoy immediately.

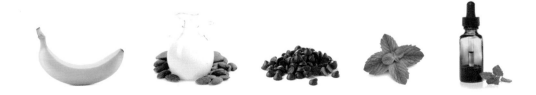

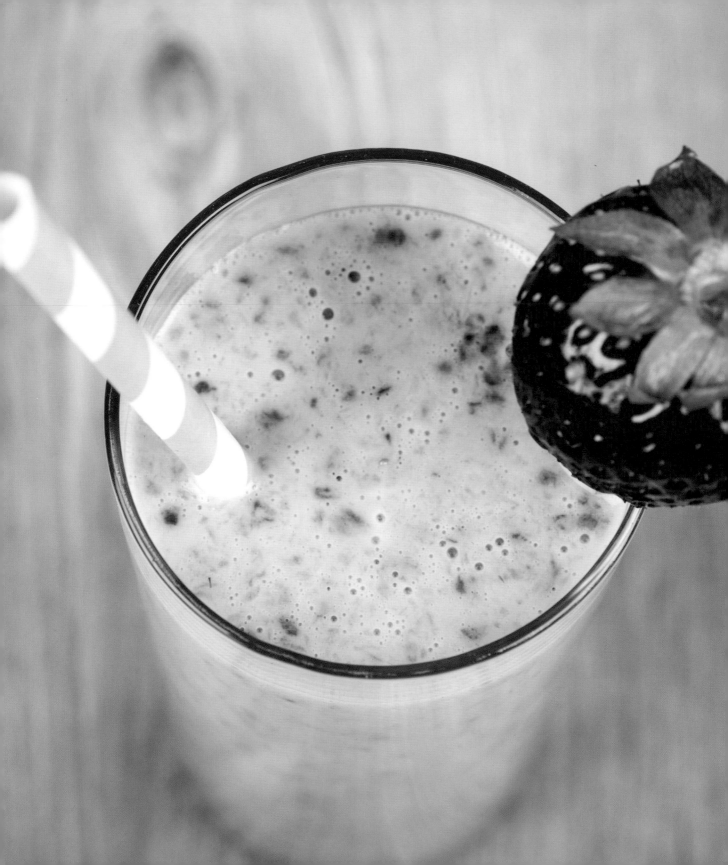

Strawberry Shortcake Smoothie

Sweet strawberry shortcake in smoothie form? Sounds delicious, doesn't it? Enjoy this healthy smoothie (guilt-free) whenever the craving strikes!

1 cup frozen strawberries

1.25 cup vanilla soy milk

1 scoop (25g) your choice of vanilla protein powder

½ tsp vanilla extract

Combine ingredients in a blender until smooth. Pour into a glass, garnish with a fresh strawberry if you'd like, and enjoy immediately.

Try this: Love chocolate-covered strawberries? Use chocolate soy milk instead of vanilla soy milk.

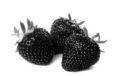

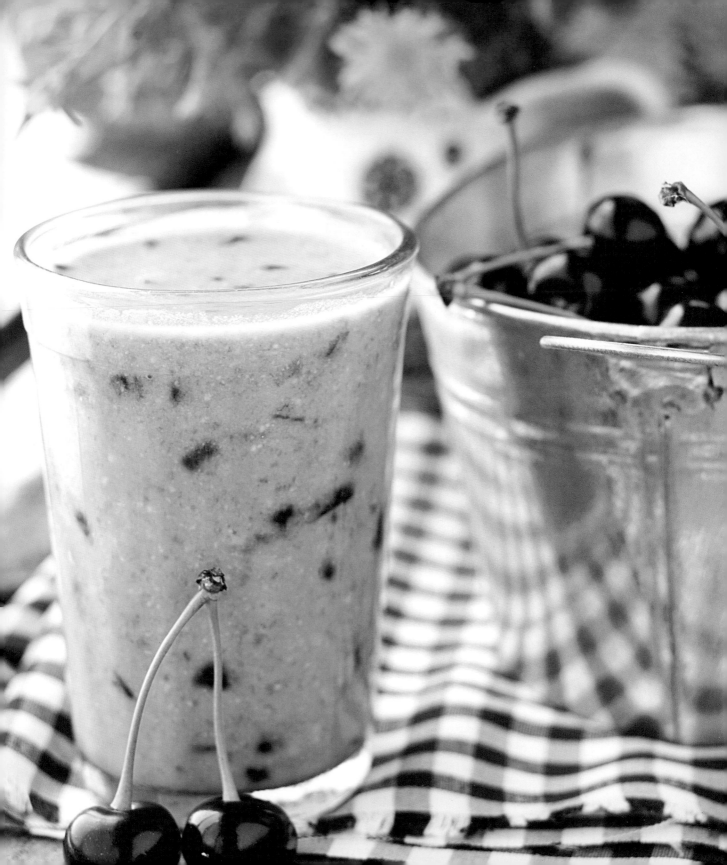

Cherry-Vanilla Smoothie

Sweet and creamy, you'll love enjoying cherries this way. A serving of yogurt adds creaminess and flavor along with some healthy fats and protein to keep you satisfied.

1 cup frozen cherries (without pits)

6 ounces yogurt (preferably vanilla-flavored)

½ cup vanilla almond milk

½ tsp vanilla extract

Combine ingredients in a blender until smooth. Pour into a glass and enjoy immediately.

Try this: For an even thicker and more satisfying smoothie, add ¼ cup of rolled oats along with an additional ½ cup of almond milk before blending.

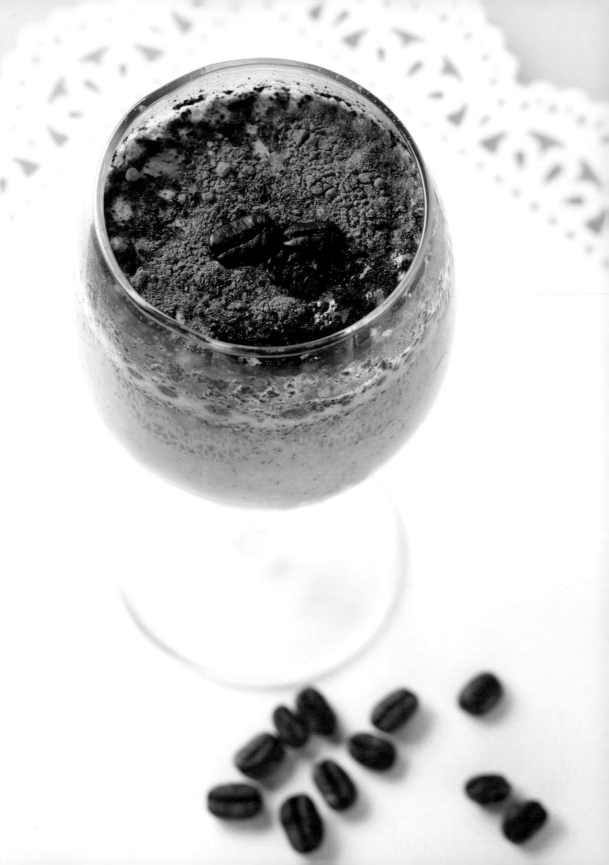

Iced Mocha Smoothie

Iced mochas are sure delicious, but they're typically loaded with sugar and high in calories. This one is figure-friendly, is nutritious, and tastes just as delicious—if not better—than the original!

1 frozen banana

2 Medjool dates

½ cup iced coffee

¾ cup chocolate almond milk

¼ tsp vanilla extract

4 ice cubes

Cinnamon to taste (optional)

Combine ingredients in a blender until smooth. Pour into a glass and serve immediately.

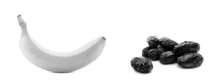

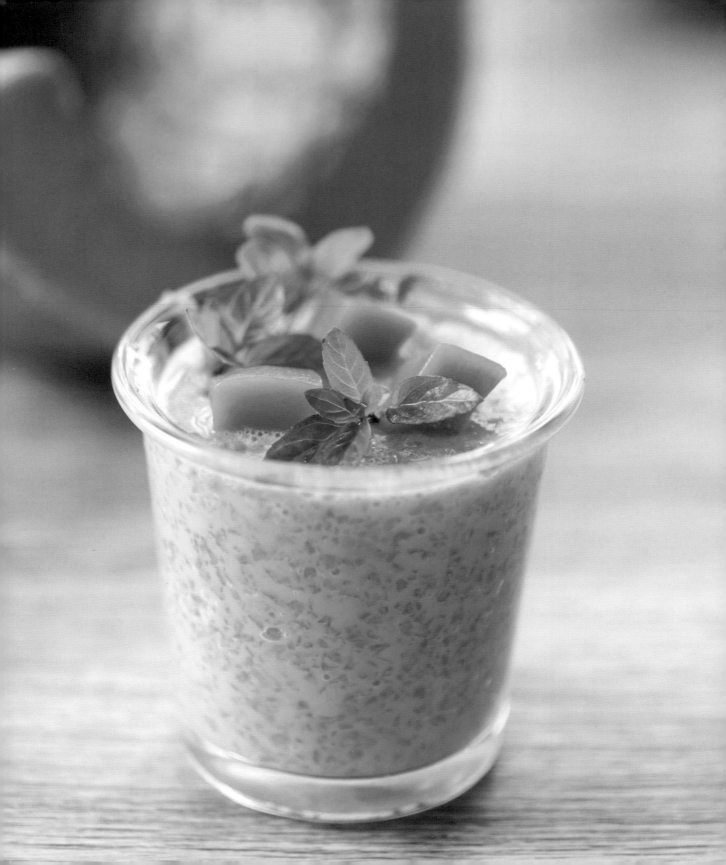

Pumpkin Pie Smoothie

Pumpkin pie all year long? You bet! This smoothie is loaded with vitamin-rich pumpkin and soymilk as well as satisfying Greek yogurt, so it's healthier than the holiday dessert.

½ cup canned pumpkin puree

½ frozen banana

6 ounces Greek yogurt (vanilla)

¾ cup vanilla soy milk

1 tbsp maple syrup

2 tsp pumpkin pie spice

½ tsp vanilla extract

4–5 ice cubes

2 tablespoons of chopped walnuts (optional)

Combine ingredients in a blender until smooth. Pour into a glass and enjoy immediately.

> *"Vegetables are a must on a diet. I suggest carrot cake, zucchini bread, and pumpkin pie."*
>
> **—JIM DAVIS**

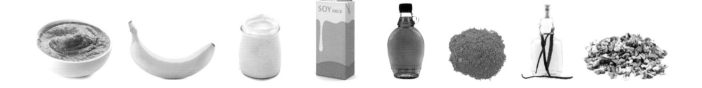

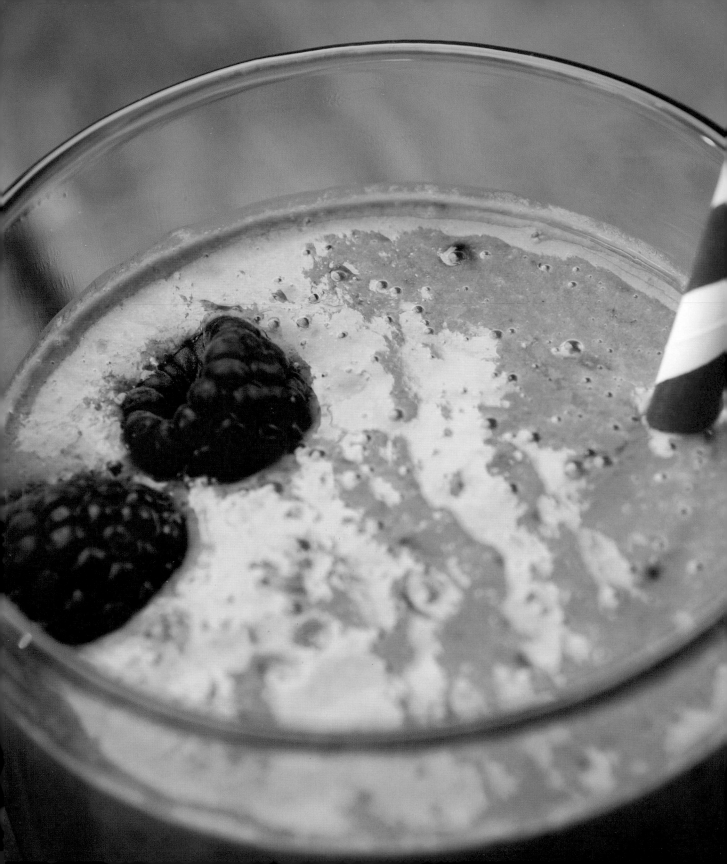

Raspberries & Cream

Raspberries and cream... so simple, so delicious, and so easy to enjoy in smoothie form. Made with just three ingredients, this smoothie makes healthy eating simple and oh so delicious!

1 cup frozen raspberries

1.25 cup vanilla soy milk

1 scoop (20g) your choice of **vanilla** protein powder

Combine ingredients in a blender until smooth. Pour into a glass and enjoy immediately.

> **Raspberries are high in fiber, vitamin C, potassium and folate. They can also help lower blood pressure and have anti-inflammatory properties that may help to reduce inflammation of the joints.**

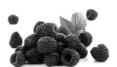

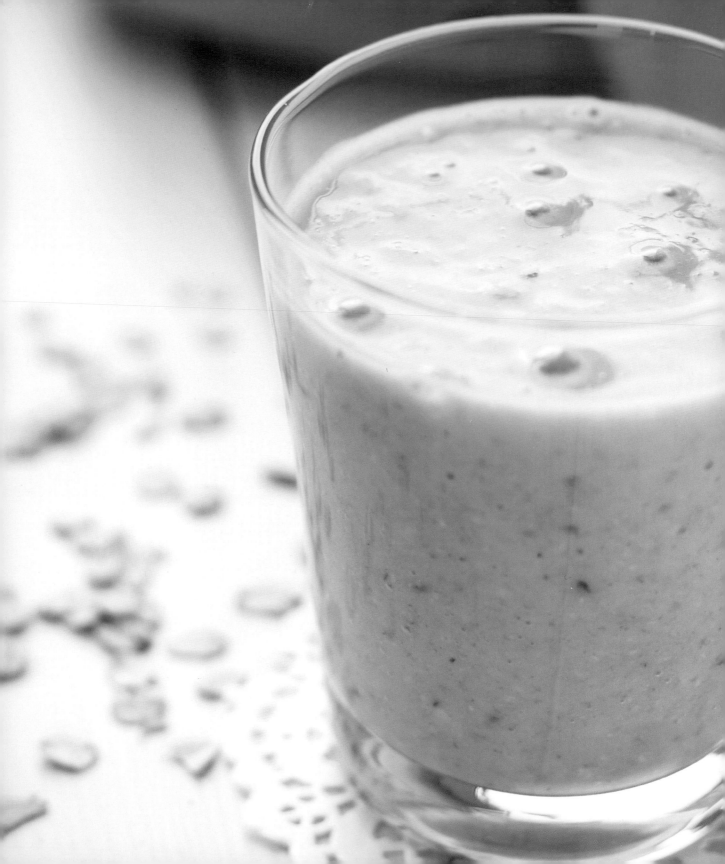

Oatmeal Raisin Cookie Smoothie

If you've ever wanted to eat cookies for breakfast, this recipe is for you! Rolled oats, banana, Medjool dates, and vanilla-flavored almond milk combine for this delightful dessert smoothie.

1 frozen banana

¼ cup rolled oats

4 Medjool dates, pitted

1.25 cups vanilla almond milk

½ tsp vanilla extract

½ tsp cinnamon

2 tsp honey (or agave nectar)

Pinch of sea salt

Combine ingredients in a blender until smooth. Pour into a glass and enjoy immediately.

Try this: For a Chocolate Oatmeal Cookie Smoothie, replace the vanilla almond milk with 1.25 cups of chocolate almond milk.

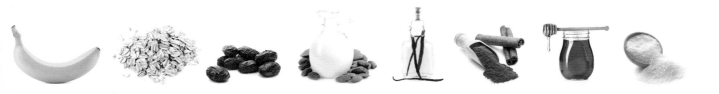

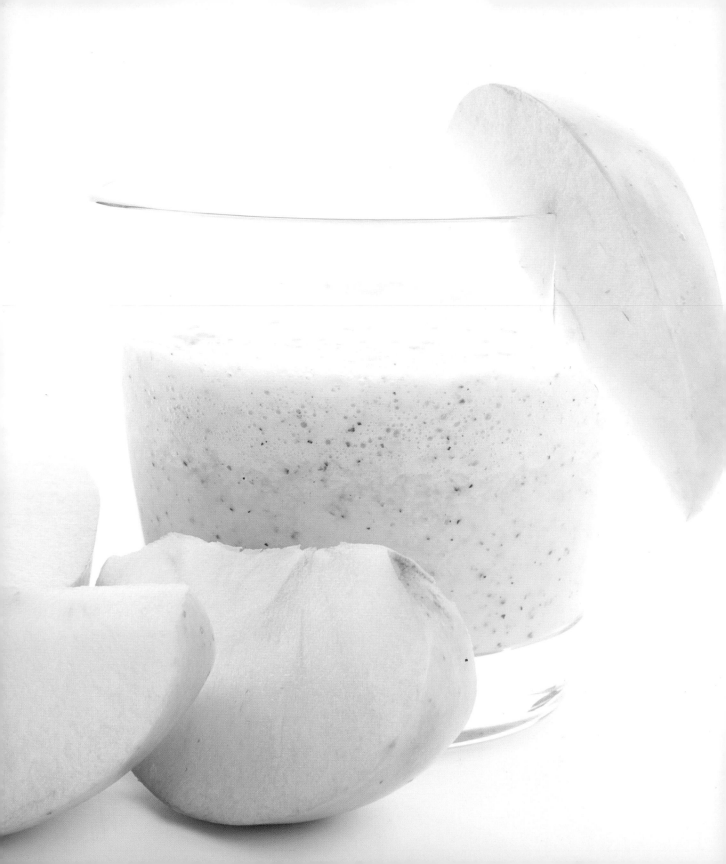

Apple Pie Smoothie

Apple pie year-round? You bet! This seasonal treat can be enjoyed all year long and for a fraction of the calories and fat. Indulge guilt-free.

1 apple, cored and diced

½ frozen banana

¼ cup cashews

2 Medool dates, pitted

1 cup vanilla almond milk

1 scoop your choice of vanilla protein powder

½ tsp cinnamon

4–5 ice cubes

Combine ingredients in a blender until smooth. Pour into a glass and enjoy immediately.

> *"If you wish to make an apple pie from scratch, you must first invent the universe."*
>
> —CARL SAGAN

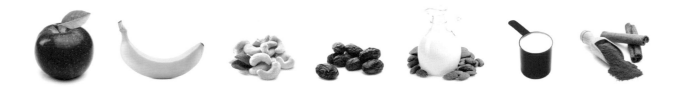

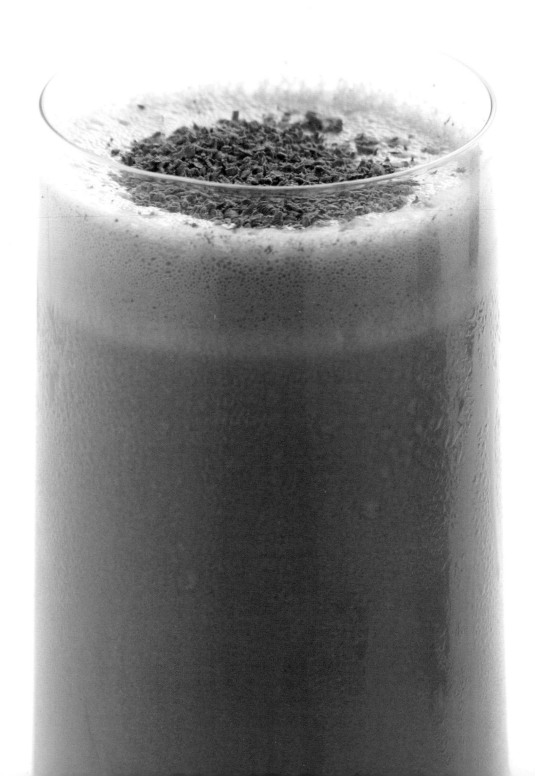

Peanut Butter Cup Smoothie

There's nothing better than the combination of peanut butter and chocolate. And what better way to combine them in a cool, creamy smoothie?

1.5 frozen banana

1.5 cup chocolate soy milk

2–3 tbsp peanut butter

Combine ingredients in a blender until smooth. Pour into a glass and enjoy immediately.

Bananas provide a healthy dose of potassium, which is essential for replenishing electrolytes that are lost through sweat during exercise.

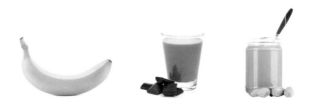

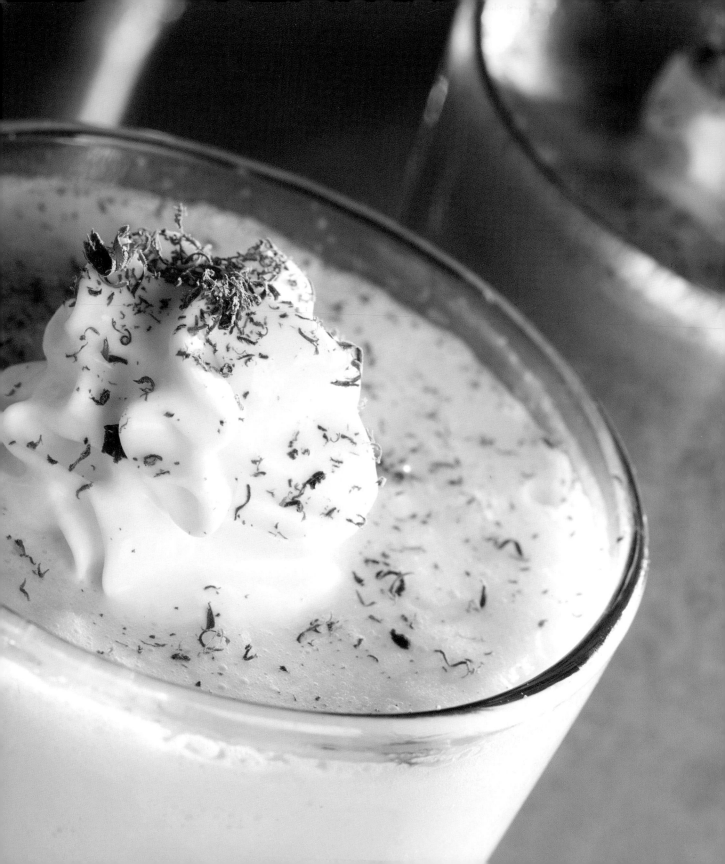

Almond Joy Smoothie

Sweet coconut, nutty almond, and rich chocolate are already an incredible flavor combination, but when mixed in a cold, creamy smoothie? Totally *irresistible!*

1.25 cups vanilla almond milk

4 Medjool dates, pitted

2 tbsp creamy almond butter

1 tbsp coconut butter, softened

1 tbsp shredded coconut

2 tbsp chocolate chips (or vegan-approved chocolate morsels)

4–5 ice cubes

Combine ingredients in a blender until smooth. Pour into a glass and enjoy immediately.

Try this: Sometimes you feel like a nut, sometimes you don't! Feel free to omit the almond butter from this recipe.

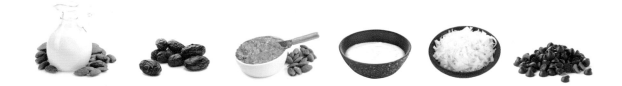

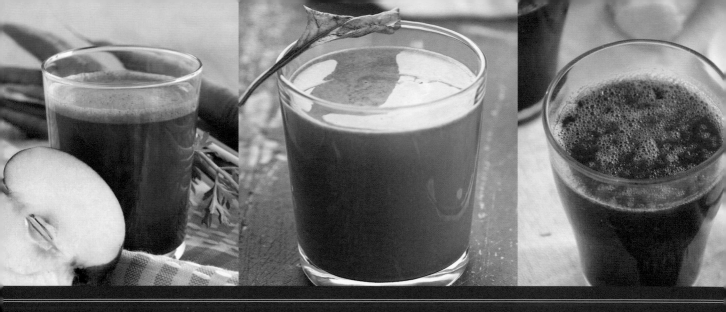

Chapter 7

Simple Juices

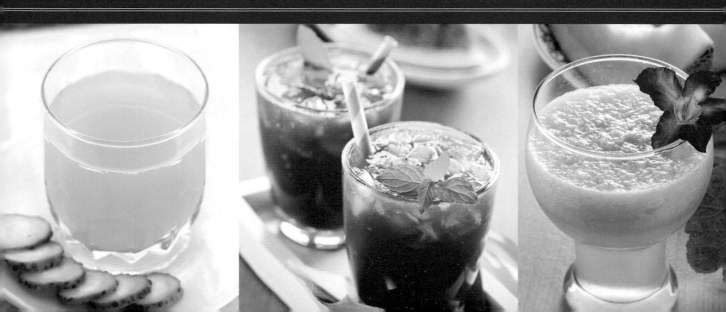

The best part about making freshly pressed juice is that it can be so simple. Even the juice of a single vegetable or fruit is a tasty and healthy addition to your diet.

Most of the recipes in this chapter have just three ingredients, so you can juice them up in a matter of minutes and still reap the health benefits of freshly pressed juice from nutrient-rich produce.

You'll find traditional juice staples such as apple, orange, grape, pear, lemon, grapefruit, and cranberry. But this chapter also includes some ingredients you may not have tried in juice before, such as cucumber, dandelion green, celery, parsley, beets, carrots, cantaloupe, and watermelon. Enjoy experimenting!

Oh, and if you're following a strict vegan diet, all the juices in this book are vegan.

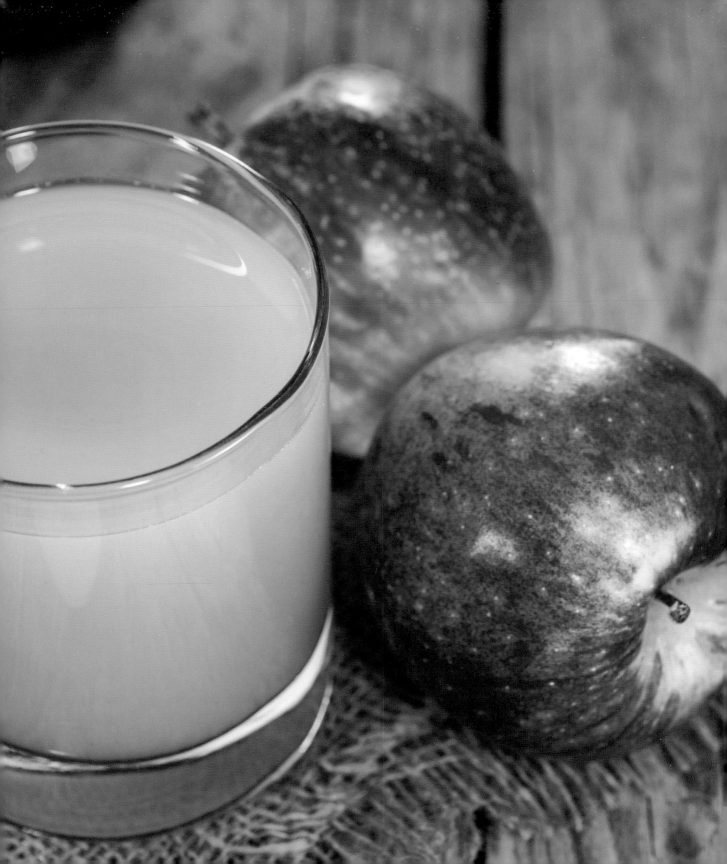

Crisp Apple Juice

Imagine biting into a fresh, right-off-the-tree apple. This juice blend tastes just like that—crisp and delicious!

2 apples
1 cup green grapes
¼ lemon

Combine all ingredients in a juicer. Pour juice into a glass or over ice and drink immediately.

> You've heard the old saying "an apple a day keeps the doctor away." Apples are rich in vitamin C, which is essential to a strong immune system. Therefore, frequently using apples in your smoothies and juices may indeed help your body fight off colds and other illnesses.

 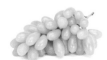

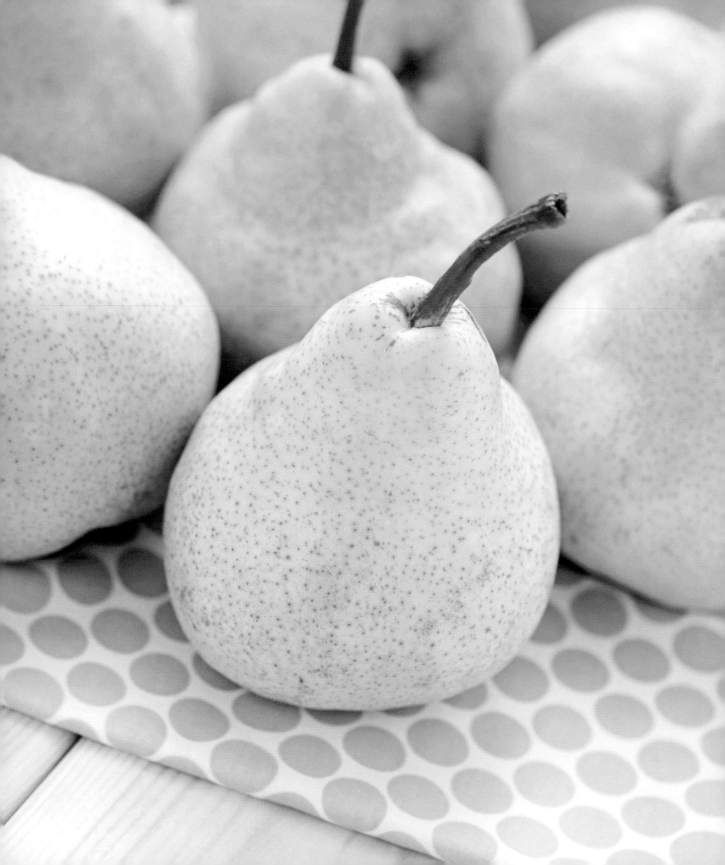

Perfect Pear Juice

Simple and nutritious, this juice comes together in matter of minutes, thanks to just three ingredients. Sweet pear combines with spinach and cucumber for a wonderful flavor and nutrient combination that you'll want to drink again and again.

3 pears
2–4 ounces spinach
½ cucumber

Put ingredients into a juicer, alternating greens with chunked fruits and veggies. Pour into a glass and drink immediately.

> Pears are a good source of vitamin C! A medium sized pear contains about 10 percent of your daily recommended value. In addition, pears are loaded with phytonutrients and antioxidants, a variety of which are found in the vibrantly colored skins.

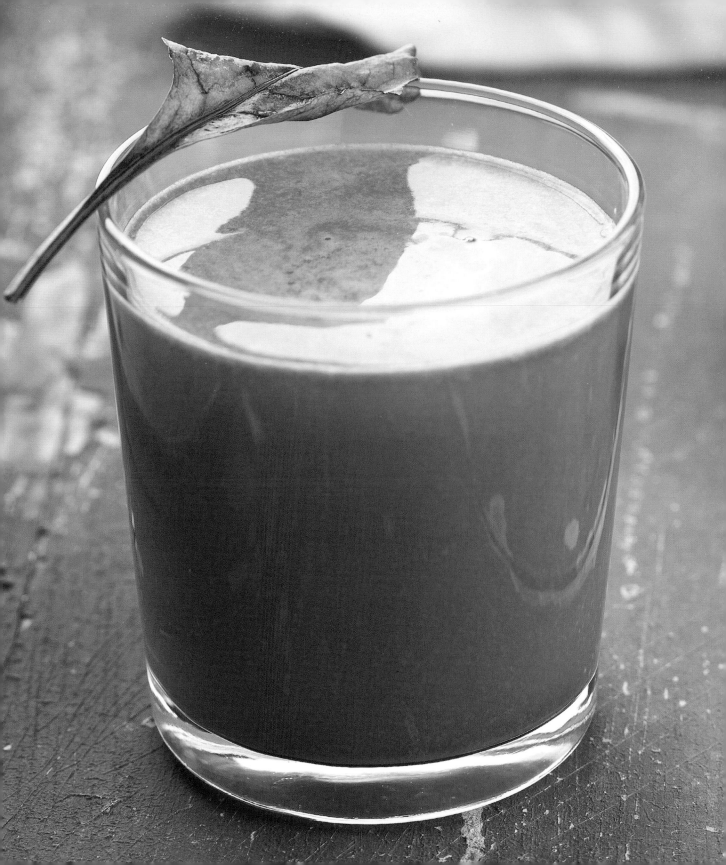

Dandy Blend

Dandelion greens are a little bitter. But when combined with sweet apple and lemon citrus, they make a refreshing, mellow, and slightly sweet green juice.

1 bunch dandelion greens
2 apples
¼ lemon

Put ingredients into a juicer, alternating greens with chunked fruits and veggies. Pour into a glass or over ice and drink immediately.

Dandelion greens are loaded with calcium and iron—even more so than other greens. In addition, they have more protein per serving than spinach.

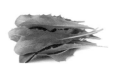

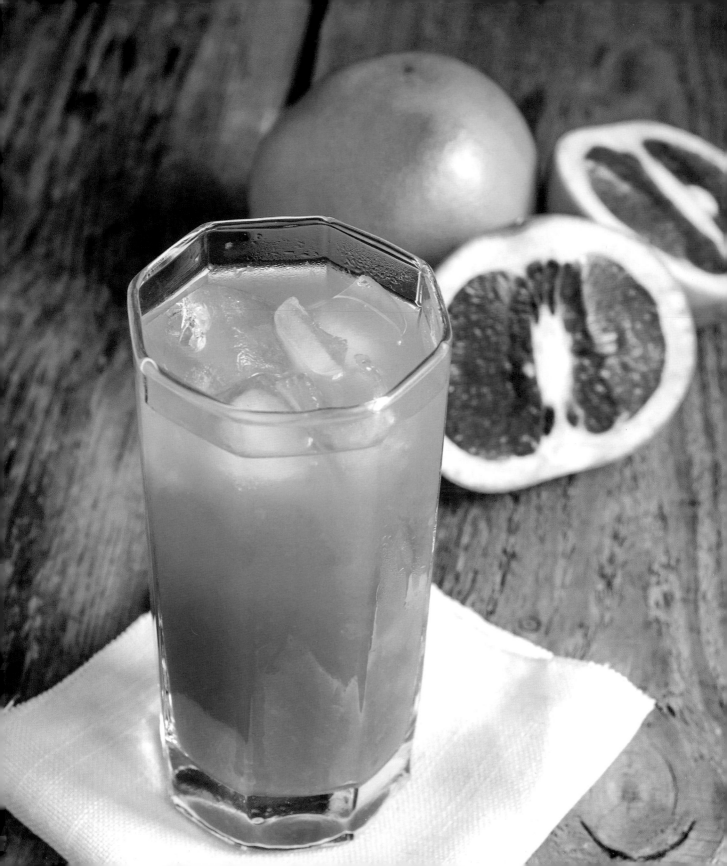

Grapefruit-Carrot-Ginger Juice

Citrus and ginger are always an exciting flavor combination. This juice takes it one step further with sweet, earthy carrot.

1 pink grapefruit, peeled and sectioned
6 carrots
Fresh ginger root to taste

Combine all ingredients in a juicer. Pour juice into a glass or over ice and drink immediately.

"A grapefruit is a lemon that had a chance and took advantage of it."

—OSCAR WILDE

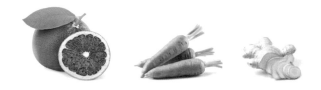

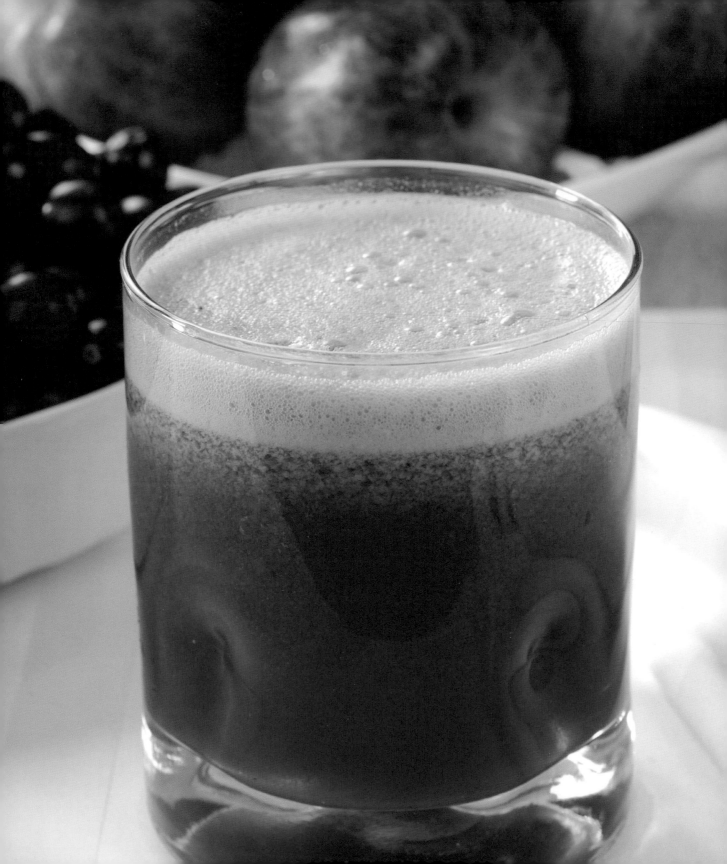

Cran-Apple-Orange Juice

Tart cranberries combine with sweet apple and orange for a tangy juice blend that you will love. Cranberries are a good source of vitamin C, E, and fiber as well as dental health.

2 apples
1 orange
1 cup cranberries

Combine all ingredients in a juicer. Pour juice into a glass or over ice and drink immediately.

Try this: Instead of an orange, substitute 1 cup of fresh strawberries.

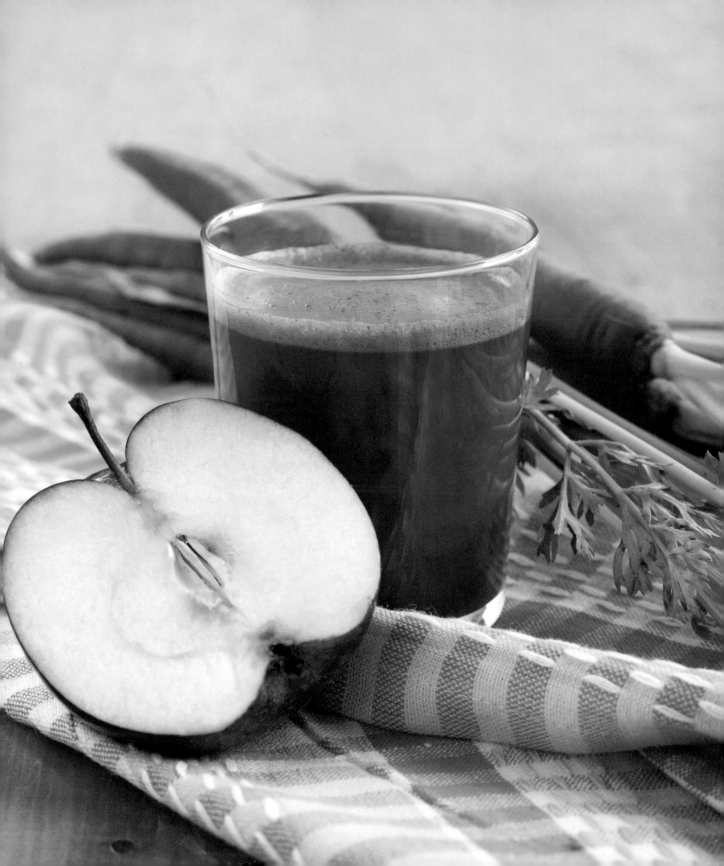

Carrot-Apple-Celery Juice

Carrots and celery combine with sweet apple for this well-balanced juice combo. Fresh parsley adds a slightly peppery flavor.

1 apple (or pear)

4 carrots

4 celery stalks

½ bunch of flat-leaf parsley (optional)

Combine all ingredients in a juicer. Pour juice into a glass or over ice and drink immediately.

Try this: For a spicy-sour kick, add freshly grated ginger root and the juice of half of a lemon.

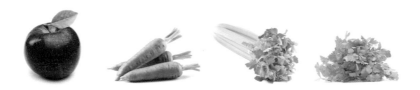

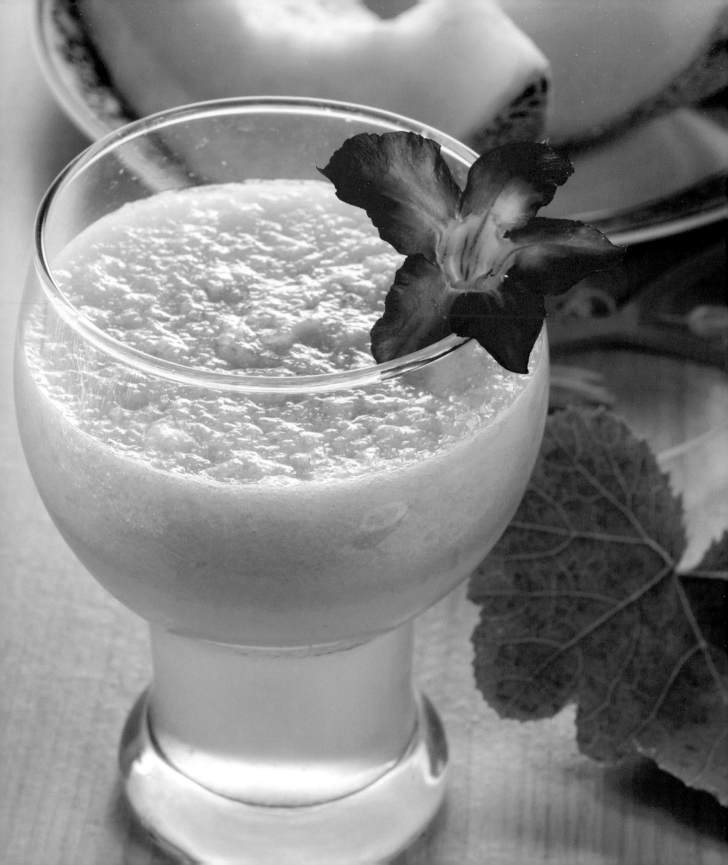

Cantaloupe-Ginger Juice

Smooth and sweet with a hint of gingery spice, this juice is both hydrating and packed with vitamin A and C.

1 cantaloupe, cut into chunks
Fresh ginger root to taste
¼ lemon (optional)

Combine all ingredients in a juice. Pour juice into a glass or over ice and drink immediately.

Do you leave your cantaloupe on the kitchen counter to ripen? You might be surprised to hear that cantaloupe does not ripen after it is picked. Once it's removed from the vine it will not sweeten any further, so there's no need to wait to cut into it.

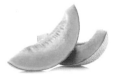

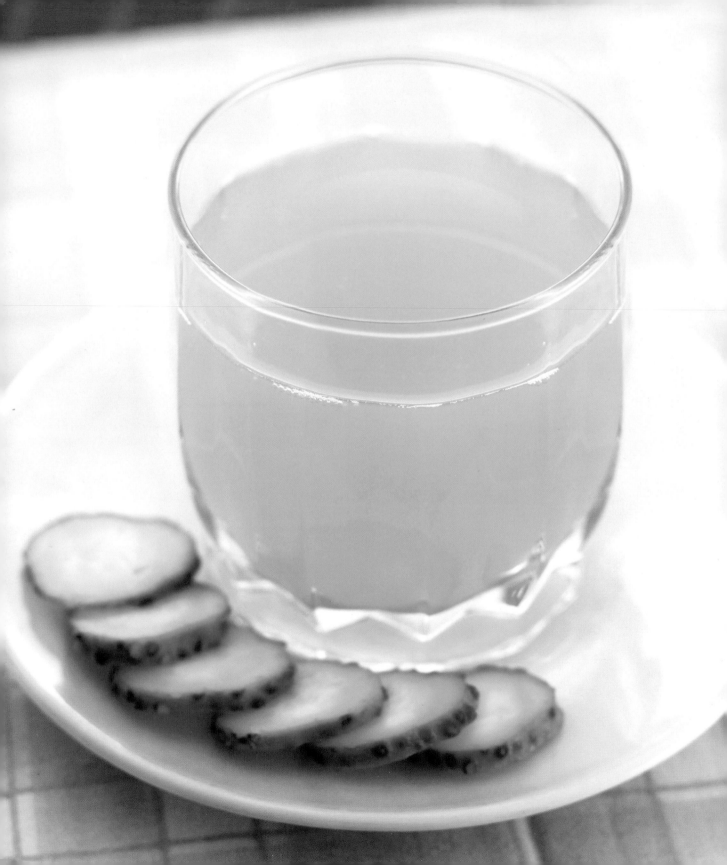

Cucumber Cooler

This Cucumber Cooler is sweet and refreshing. Cucumbers are a natural pick-me-up. They're a good source of B vitamins, which give you energy, and hydrate your body (cucumbers are 95 percent water) helping it eliminate toxins at the same time.

1 apple
1 cucumber
1 cup green grapes

Combine all ingredients in a juicer. Pour juice into a glass or over ice and drink immediately.

Try this: Add 8–10 fresh mint leaves before blending.

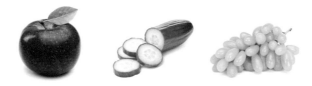

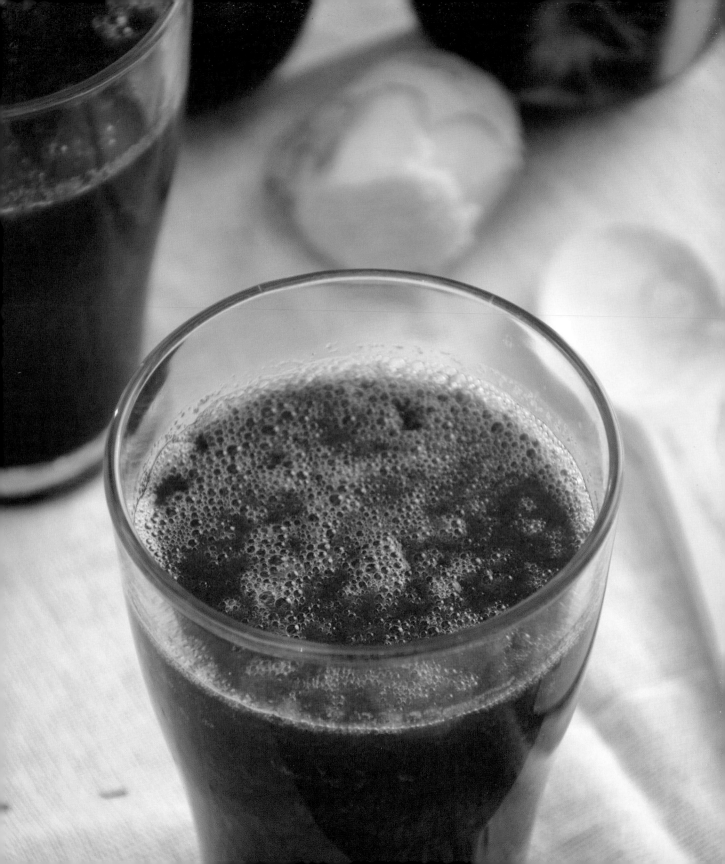

ABP (Apple-Beet-Pear) Juice

Simple and delicious, this juice blend combines the flavors of earthy beets with sweet apple and pear and sour lemon to keep your taste buds guessing!

1 apple
1 pear
2 beets
Juice of ½ lemon
Fresh ginger root to taste (optional)

Combine all ingredients in a juicer. Pour juice into a glass or over ice and drink immediately.

> *"The beet is the most intense of vegetables. The radish, admittedly, is more feverish, but the fire of the radish is a cold fire, the fire of discontent, not of passion. Tomatoes are lusty enough, yet there runs through tomatoes an undercurrent of frivolity. Beets are deadly serious."*
>
> —TOM ROBBINS

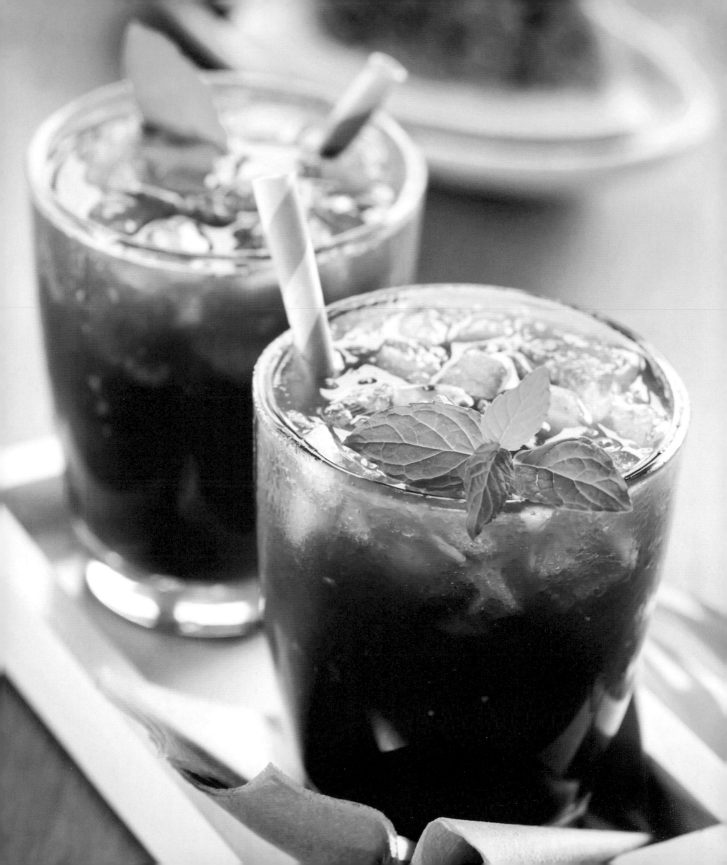

Watermelon-Cantaloupe Cooler

In the middle of a hot, humid summer, you will love this simple, cool, and refreshing juice that is packed full of antioxidants and vitamins.

1 cup watermelon, cut into chunks

½ cup cantaloupe, cut into chunks

½ cucumber

Juice of ¼ lemon (optional)

Combine all ingredients in a juicer. Pour juice into a glass over ice and drink immediately.

> *"When one has tasted watermelon he knows what the angels eat."*
>
> —MARK TWAIN

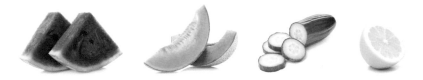

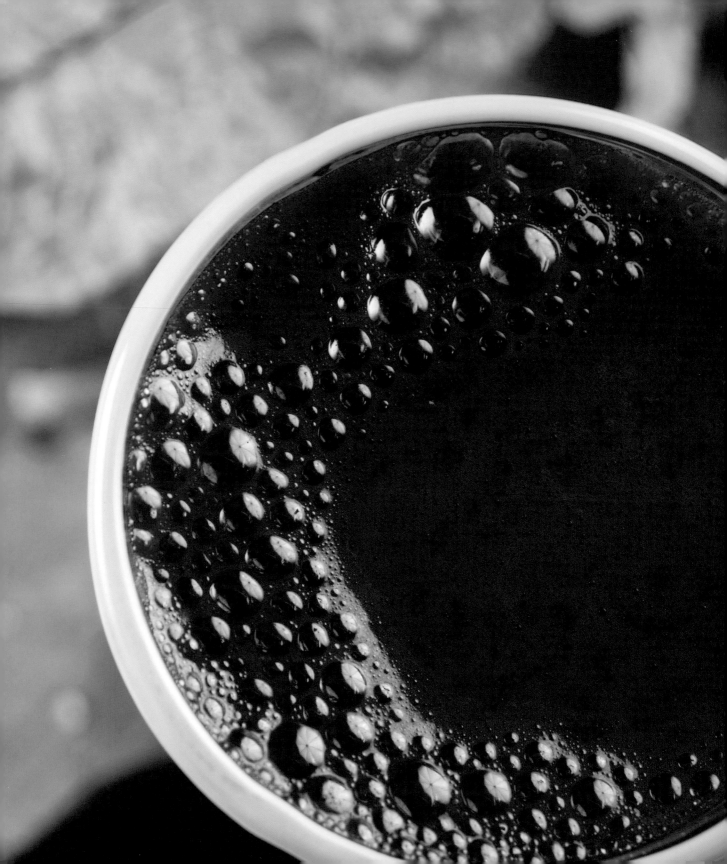

V3 Juice

Made with just three different vegetables, this simple juice comes together in a matter of minutes and, boy, does it pack a nutritional punch. Packed with vitamin A, C, folate, fiber, and whole slew of antioxidants, this juice will make you feel a tad bit healthier starting with the very first sip.

2 beets
5 carrots
1 cucumber

Combine all ingredients in a juicer. Pour juice into a glass or over ice and drink immediately.

> *"Eat food. Not too much. Mostly plants."*
> —MICHAEL POLLAN

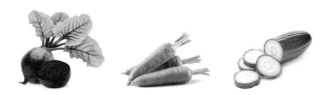

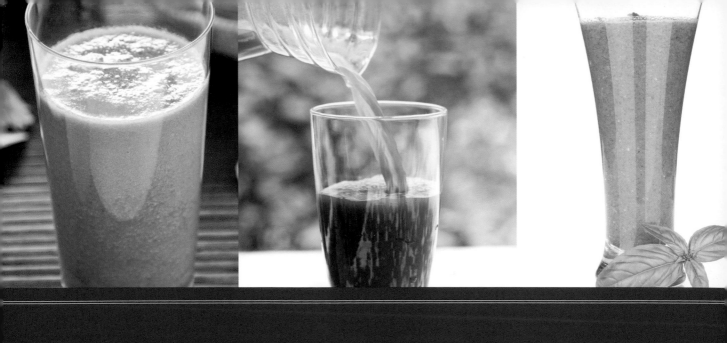

Chapter 8

Green Juices

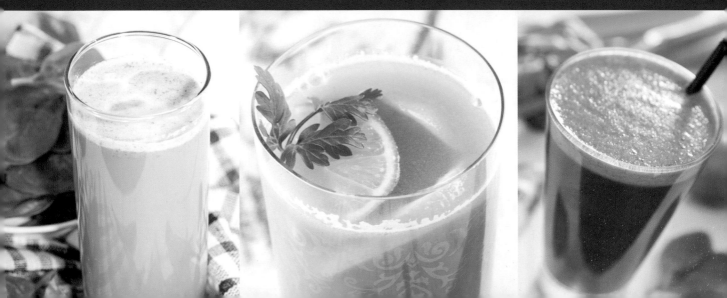

We've all heard it before: Fill your diet with leafy greens to reap the health benefits, because, calorie for calories, they're one of the most concentrated sources of nutrition of any foods. One easy way to ensure that you're getting these essential vitamins, minerals, and disease-fighting phytochemicals in your diet is by juicing them.

The juice recipes in this chapter have one obvious thing in common: they're green. Less obvious is how truly nutritious they are for you. Leafy greens—the darker the better—are a rich source of minerals, including iron, calcium, potassium, and magnesium and vitamins, including vitamins K, C, E, and many of the B vitamins. In addition, they provide a variety of phytonutrients and even small amounts of omega-3 fats. With such a wealth of health in one glass, it's no wonder the green juice trend has caught on. It's an incredibly healthy way to boost your vitality and wellness. Bottoms up!

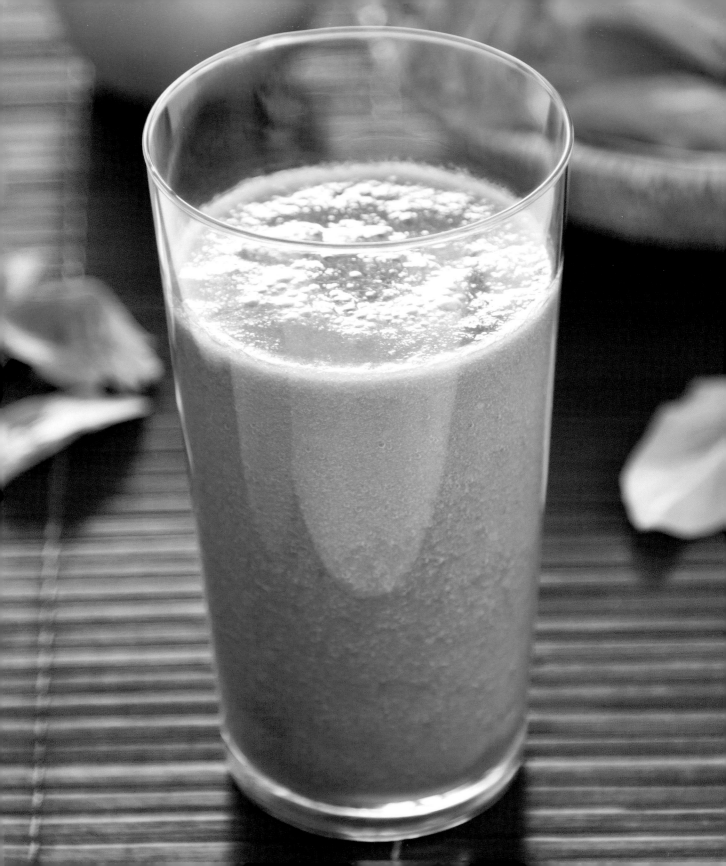

Everyday Green Juice

This is my go-to green juice recipe. Besides being delicious, it also has a great mix of flavors and nutrients. I always feel healthier after I drink a glass of this Everyday Green Juice.

4 ounces of fresh spinach or kale
1 apple
1 cucumber
4 celery stalks
Fresh ginger root to taste (optional)

Put ingredients into a juicer, alternating greens with chunked fruits and veggies. Pour into a glass or over ice and drink immediately.

> **Celery supplies essential vitamins A, C, and K as well as the minerals folic acid and potassium, which helps regulate blood pressure.**

Try this: For a citrusy kick, add the juice of a quarter or half of a lemon or lime.

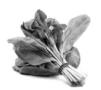

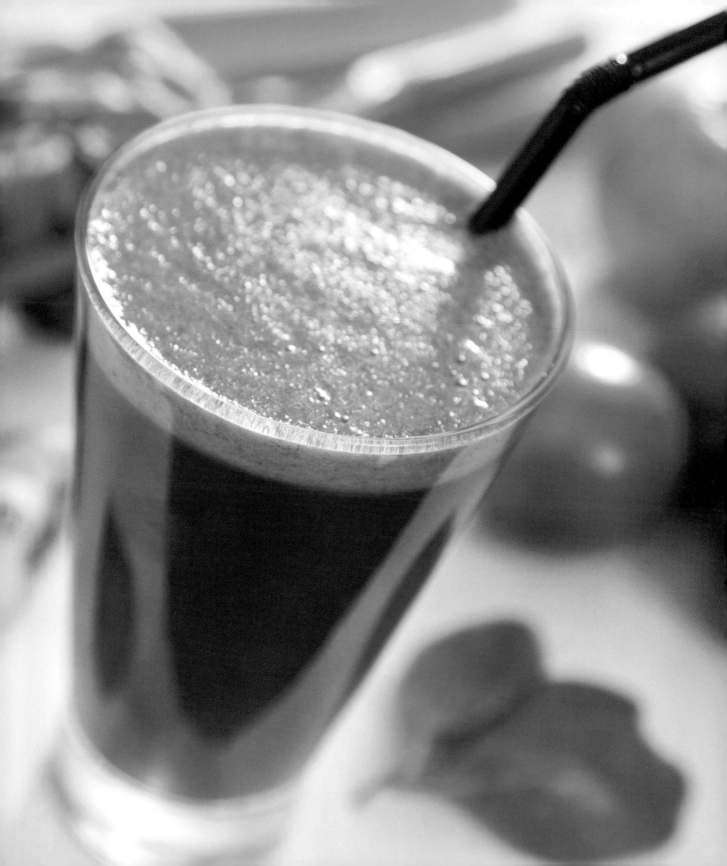

Green Citrus Juice

The ingredients in this mellow, green juice are straight-forward. But you'll be thoroughly impressed by their simple, refreshing flavors. This one is guaranteed to be a favorite.

2 ounces baby spinach
1 Granny Smith apple
¼ pink grapefruit
6 celery stalks

Put ingredients into a juicer, alternating greens with chunked fruits and veggies. Pour into a glass or over ice and drink immediately.

Try this: For a little kick, add fresh ginger root to taste.

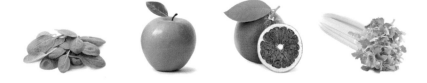

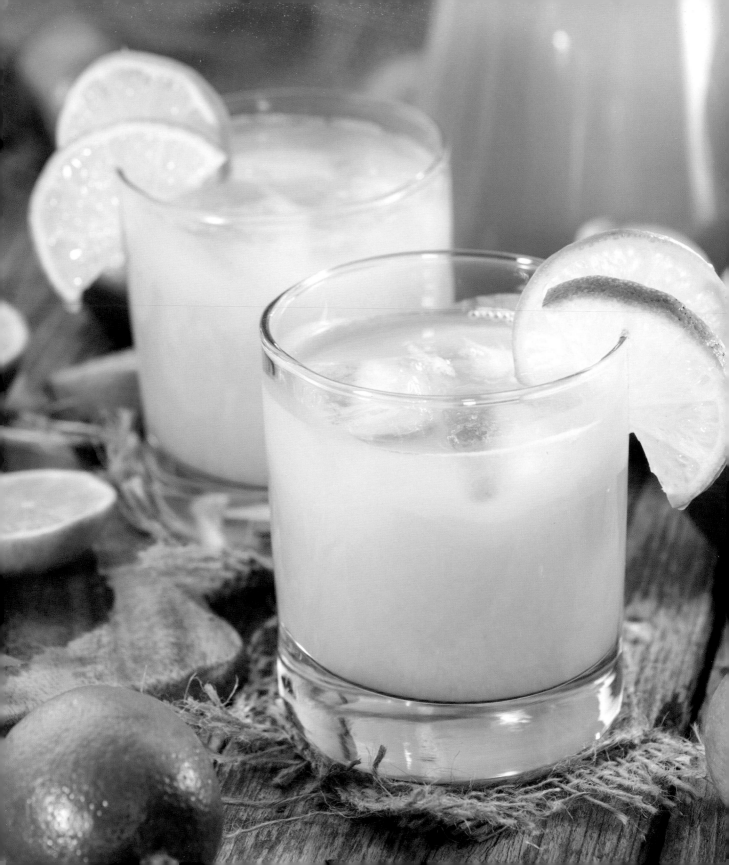

Mint-Apple-Lime Juice

There are so many wonderful flavors in this juice. Sweet, sour, bitter, refreshing... this Mint-Apple-Lime Juice will definitely keep your taste buds guessing!

2 apples
1 cucumber
1 handful of fresh spinach (or **other** leafy green)
½ lime
10–12 leaves of fresh mint

Put ingredients into a juicer, alternating greens with chunked fruits and veggies. Pour into a glass or over ice and drink immediately.

> *"To eat is a necessity, but to eat intelligently is an art."*
>
> —LA ROCHEFOUCAULD

 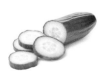

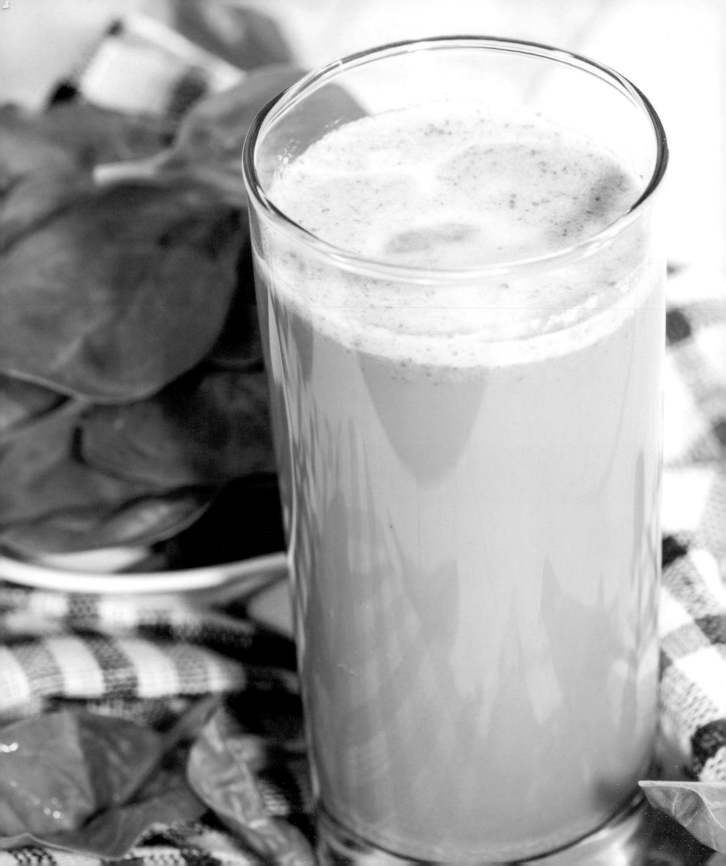

Sweet 'N' Green Juice

Sometimes bitter greens can overwhelm a juice, but fresh cantaloupe adds a subtle sweetness to this one. It's the perfect flavor balance for your taste buds.

2 ounces fresh spinach, kale or Swiss chard
½ Granny Smith apple
1 cup cubed fresh cantaloupe
1 cucumber

Put ingredients into a juicer, alternating greens with chunked fruits and veggies. Pour into a glass or over ice and drink immediately.

Try this: For a sweet and minty juice, add 8–10 leaves of fresh mint before blending.

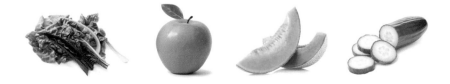

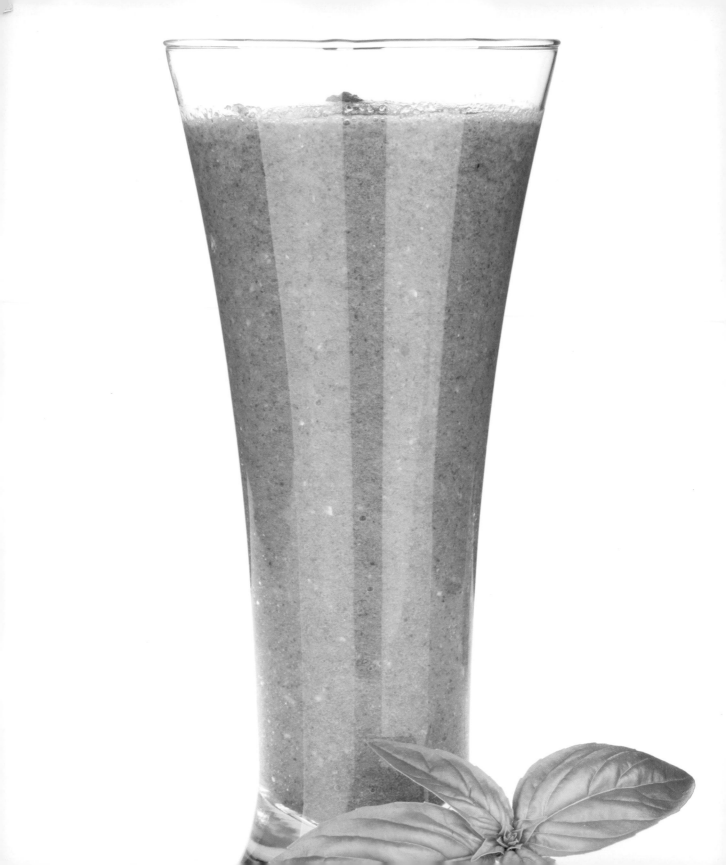

Basil-Apple-Lime Juice

The flavors in this juice will awaken all your senses. The basil is a nice complement to the sweet-tanginess of the Granny Smith apples, and the lime adds zing.

2–3 Granny Smith apples

½ cucumber

½ lime

1 bunch of basil

Combine all ingredients in a juicer. Pour juice into a glass or over ice and drink immediately.

Basil is considered one of the healthiest herbs out there. It's rich in antioxidants, vitamin A, vitamin K, vitamin C, magnesium, iron, potassium, and calcium, and it said to have anti-aging properties and help reduce inflammation and swelling.

 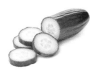

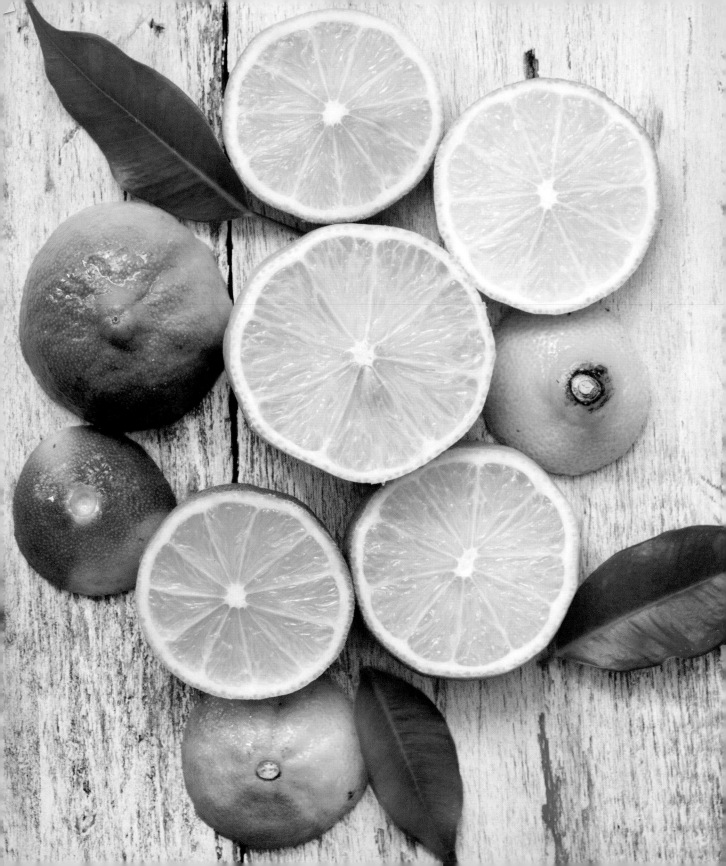

Lemon-Lime Twist Juice

The ingredients in this mellow, green juice might seem simple, but you'll be thoroughly impressed by their interesting and refreshing flavors.

2 ounces dark leafy greens of your choice
1 apple
1 lemon
1 lime
6 celery stalks

Put ingredients into a juicer, alternating greens with chunked fruits and veggies. Pour into a glass or over ice and drink immediately.

> *"Lime juice makes things taste fresher. I use it for drinks, salsas, relishes, soups, and sauces. You want some give to your limes—firmness means the inside is dry—and they'll stay softer longer if you don't refrigerate them."*
>
> —BOBBY FLAY

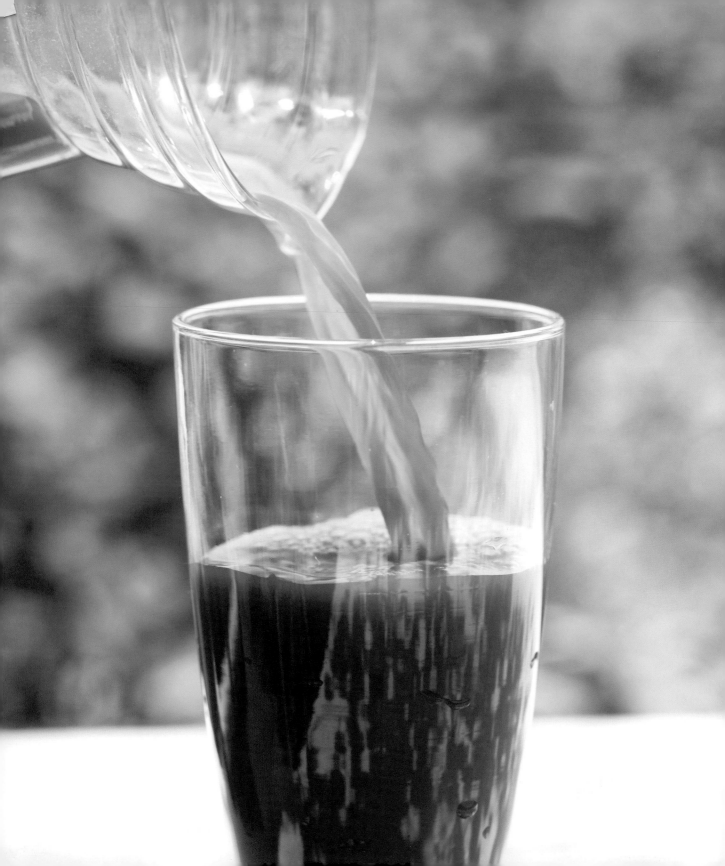

Leafy Green Goodness Juice

If you're craving some fresh greens in your diet, this juice is for you. You'll get a whole slew of antioxidants in this super green drink, loaded with kale, spinach, and Swiss chard.

2 ounces kale

2 ounces spinach

2 ounces of Swiss chard

4 celery stalks

1 cucumber

½ bunch parsley (optional)

Put ingredients into a juicer, alternating greens with chunked fruits and veggies. Pour into a glass or over ice and drink immediately.

Try this: For a sweeter version, swap out the celery stalks for a medium or large apple.

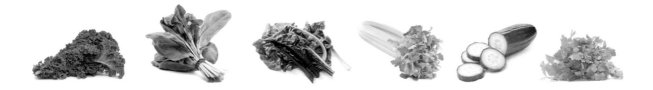

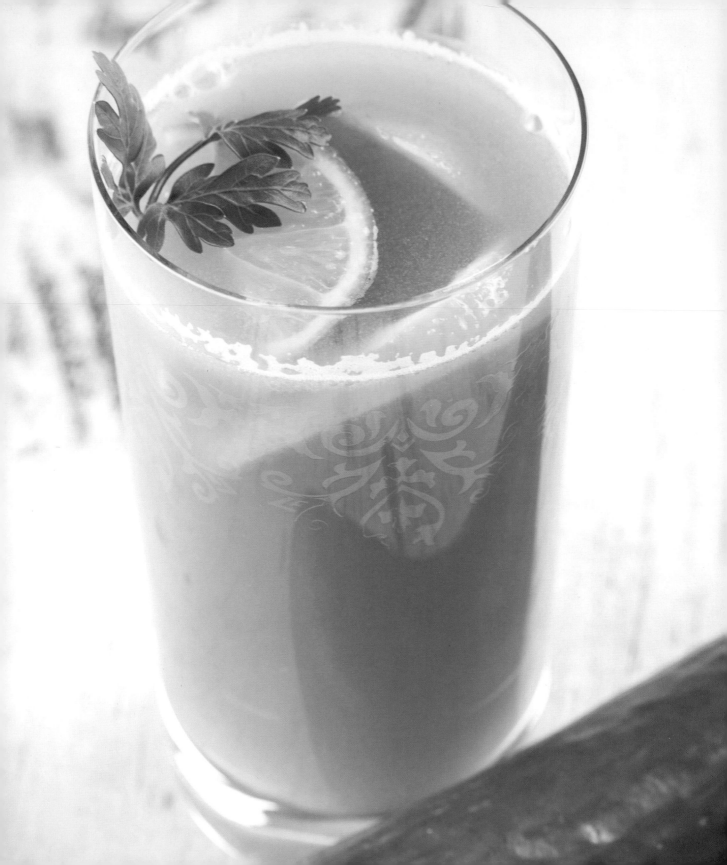

Light 'N' Green Juice

Sometimes you just feel like a light, refreshing, and hydrating green juice. Maybe dark leafy greens is a bit too bitter for your liking and you want something a little more mellow? If so, this juice is for you!

4 ounces of romaine lettuce

1 apple

1 cucumber

4 celery stalks

¼ lemon

Put ingredients into a juicer, alternating greens with chunked fruits and veggies. Pour into a glass or over ice and drink immediately.

Try this: Add a medium bunch of parsley before juicing. Finish with a few shakes of cayenne pepper and a teaspoon of hot sauce if you're feeling daring!

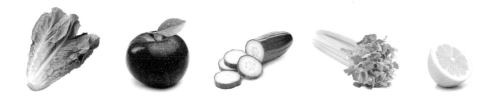

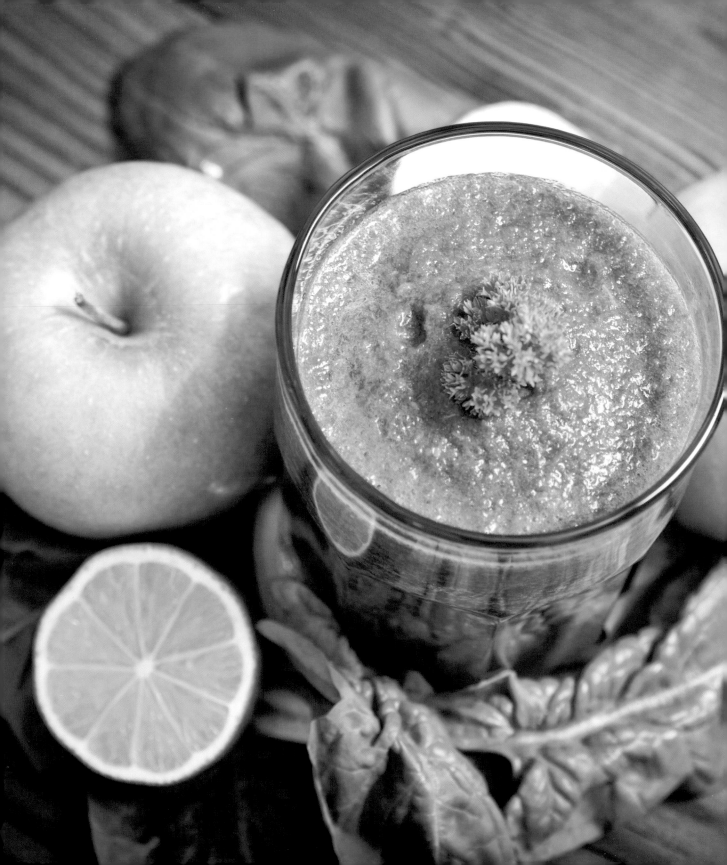

Sweet Kale Juice

Superfood kale is loaded with vitamins K, A, and C, but it's also a tad bitter-tasting. Add some apple and watermelon, though, and you've got a sweet, smooth juice.

4 ounces kale

1 apple

1 cup watermelon, cut into chunks

¼ lime (optional)

Put ingredients into a juicer, alternating greens with chunked fruits and veggies. Pour into a glass or over ice and drink immediately.

If greens such as kale or Swiss chard tend to be too bitter for you, try balancing the flavor with fresh lemon or lime. The acidity helps to neutralize the bitterness. Taste as you go: Try a good-size squeeze and then add more if needed.

 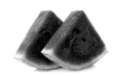

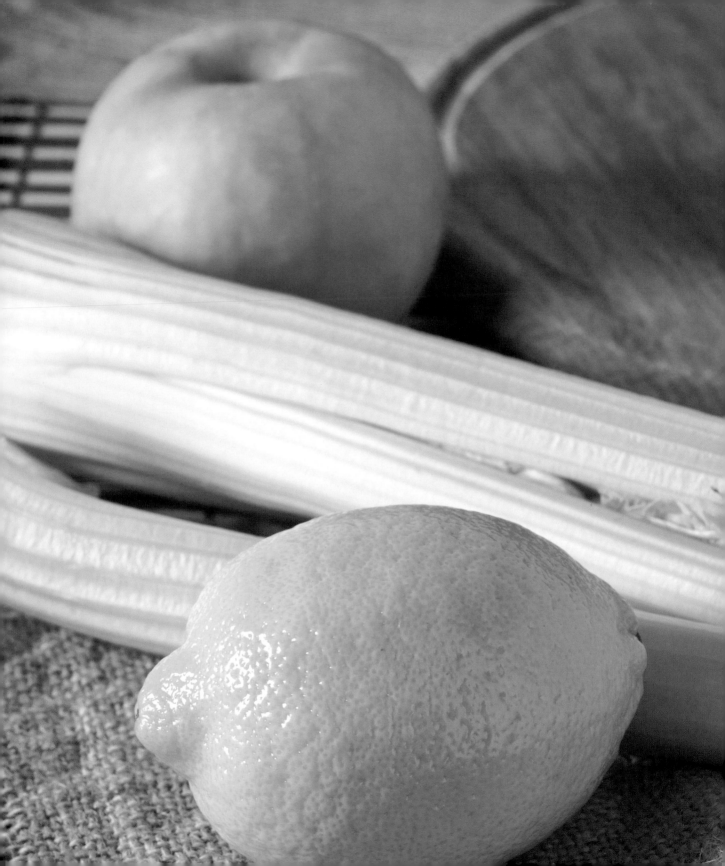

Zesty Green Ginger Juice

Looking for something to really wake you up? Perhaps something a little zesty? Here's the juice for you! Beware: It's got a little bite.

2 lemons, peeled and sliced

1 handful of spinach or kale

4 stalks of celery

½ Granny Smith apple

Fresh ginger root to taste

Put ingredients into a juicer, alternating greens with chunked fruits and veggies. Pour into a glass or over ice and drink immediately.

Try this: For a sweeter and mellower juice, replace lemons with two apples.

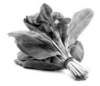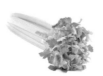

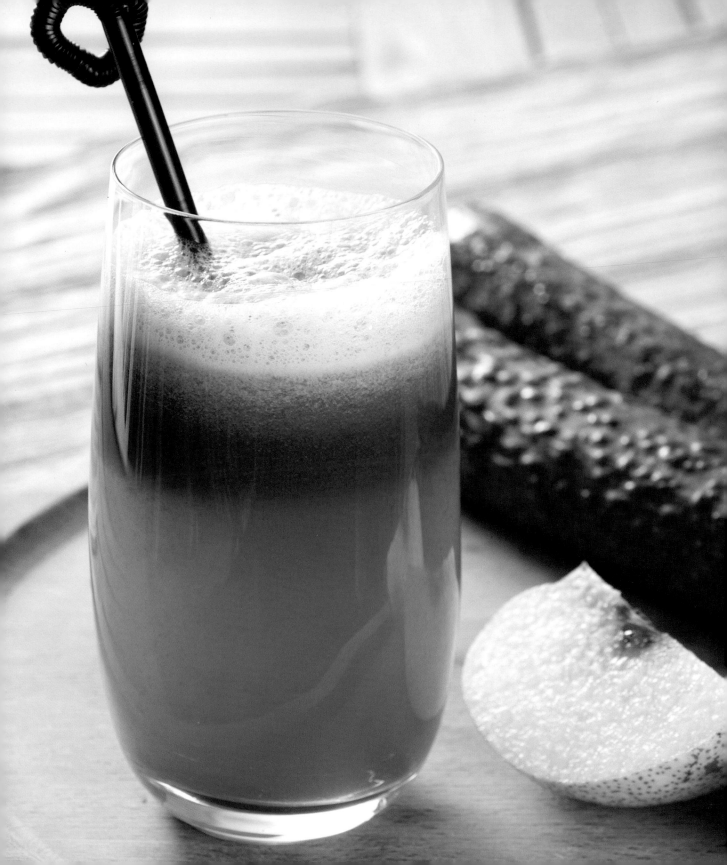

Peppery Pear Juice

There's nothing better than fresh arugula—that spicy, peppery taste is definitely something special. It combines with pear, cucumber, lemon, and ginger for a sweet, refreshing juice with a peppery zing.

4 ounces fresh arugula

1 pear

1 cucumber

½ lemon

Fresh ginger root to taste

Put ingredients into a juicer, alternating greens with chunked fruits and veggies. Pour into a glass or over ice and drink immediately.

Also known as "salad rocket," arugula is a rich source of folic acid and vitamins A and C. In addition, it's one of the best vegetable sources of vitamin K, which provides a boost for both bone and brain health.

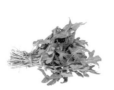

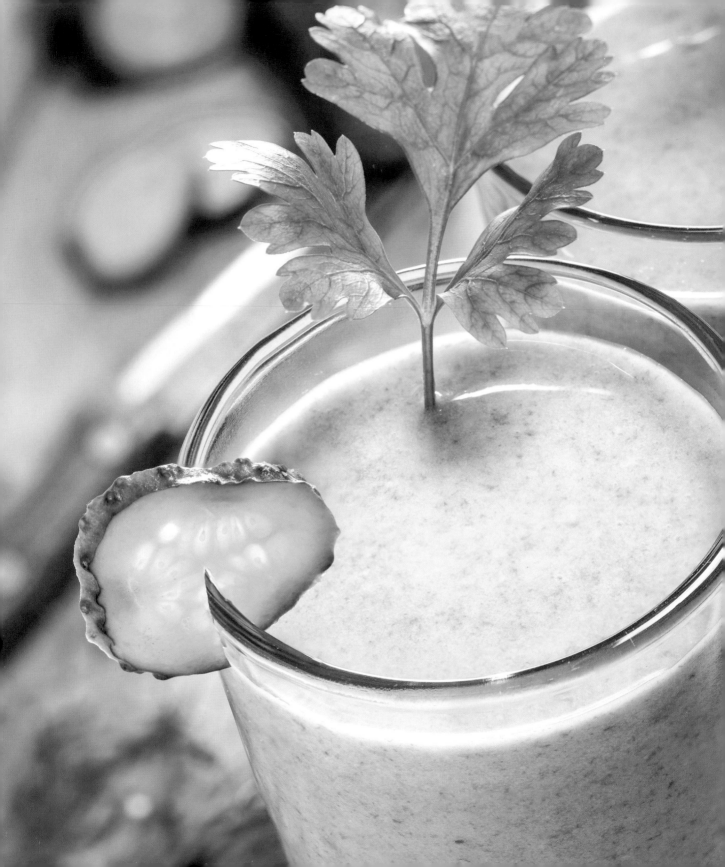

Sweet Simplicity

These five ingredients seem so simple by themselves, but when combined they create an incredibly refreshing and slightly sweet juice that you'll want to drink again and again. In fact, there's a good chance you'll want to make it part of your regular juicing rotation.

6 leaves of romaine lettuce

1 cucumber

1 apple

¼ lemon, peeled

10 mint leaves

Put ingredients into a juicer, alternating greens with chunked fruits and veggies. Pour into a glass or over ice and drink immediately.

Try this: Garnish with parsley and a cucumber slice.

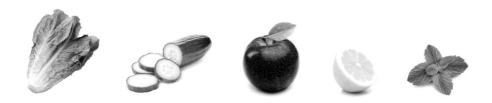

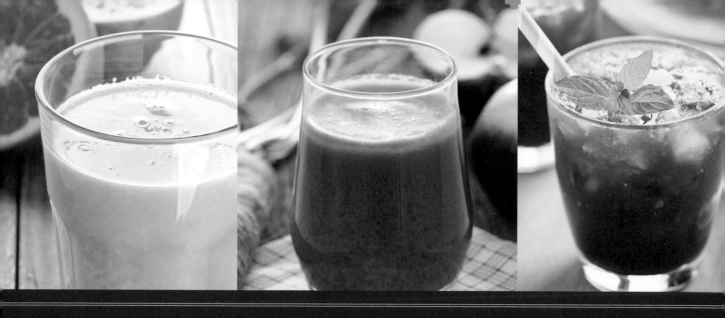

Chapter 9

Fruit Juice Blends

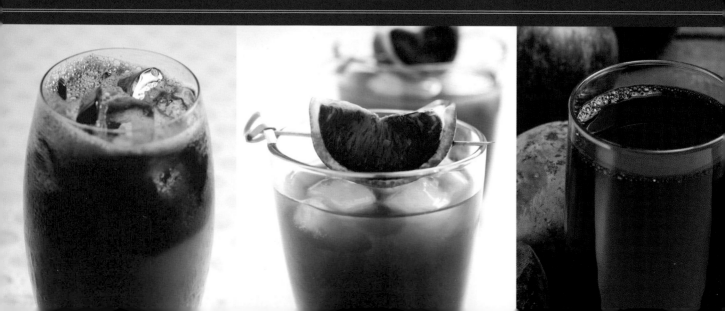

*F*ruit juice is a wonderful way to add nutrients to your diet. But most store-bought varieties aren't made with 100 percent juice and are laden with sugar or artificial sweeteners.

Making freshly pressed fruit juice is a great way to add nutrients to your diet, especially if you sneak in a few vegetables while you're at it. If you're not a big veggie eater, fruit juice blends make it easy to consume them—oftentimes without even tasting them.

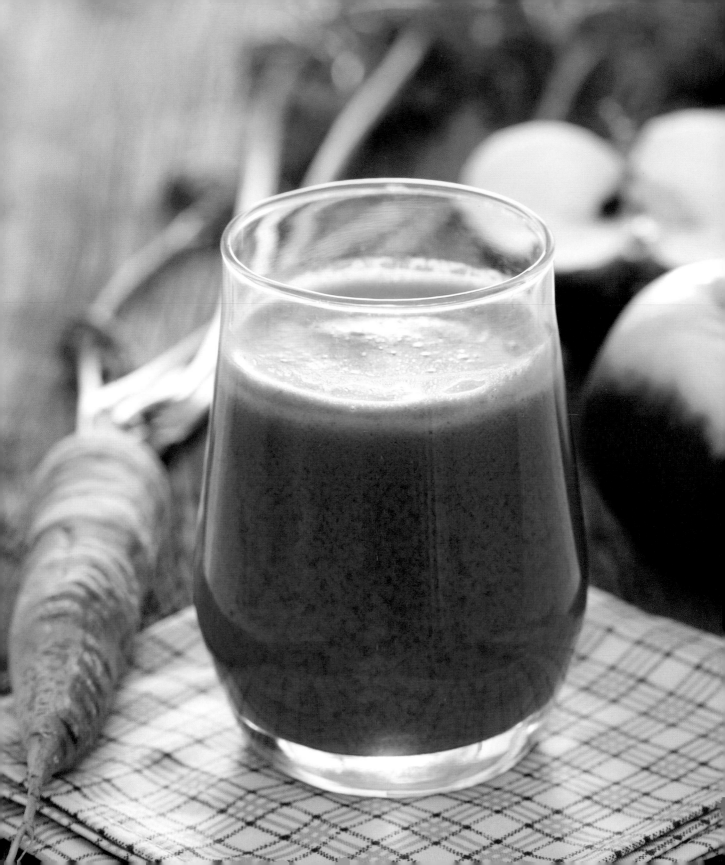

Pineapple-Ginger-Carrot Juice

This unique blend of tangy and sweet citrus juice packs a punch with a healthy dose of fresh ginger. You're guaranteed a refreshing taste experience.

½ apple
1 cup of fresh pineapple, cut into chunks
4 carrots
Fresh ginger root to taste

Combine all ingredients in a juicer. Pour juice into a glass or over ice and drink immediately.

> **Ginger is loaded with hytonutrients, which may help protect again a variety of diseases, including cancer and heart disease.**

 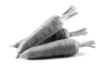

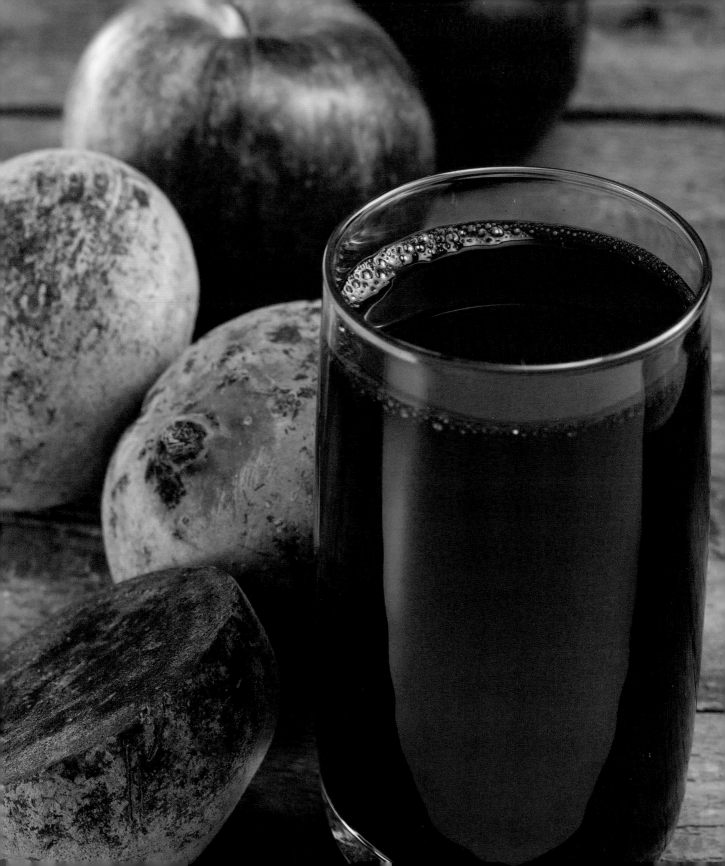

Deep Red Juice

The ingredients in this juice combine to make a beautiful deep red. It's smooth and sweet, and likely a recipe that you will return to again and again.

4 ounces spinach
1 apple
1 beet
½ cup blueberries
½ cucumber

Put ingredients into a juicer, alternating greens with chunked fruits and veggies. Pour into a glass or over ice and drink immediately.

> *"The doctor of the future will give no medicine, but will interest his patients in the care of the human frame, in a proper diet, and in the cause and prevention of disease."*
>
> —THOMAS EDISON

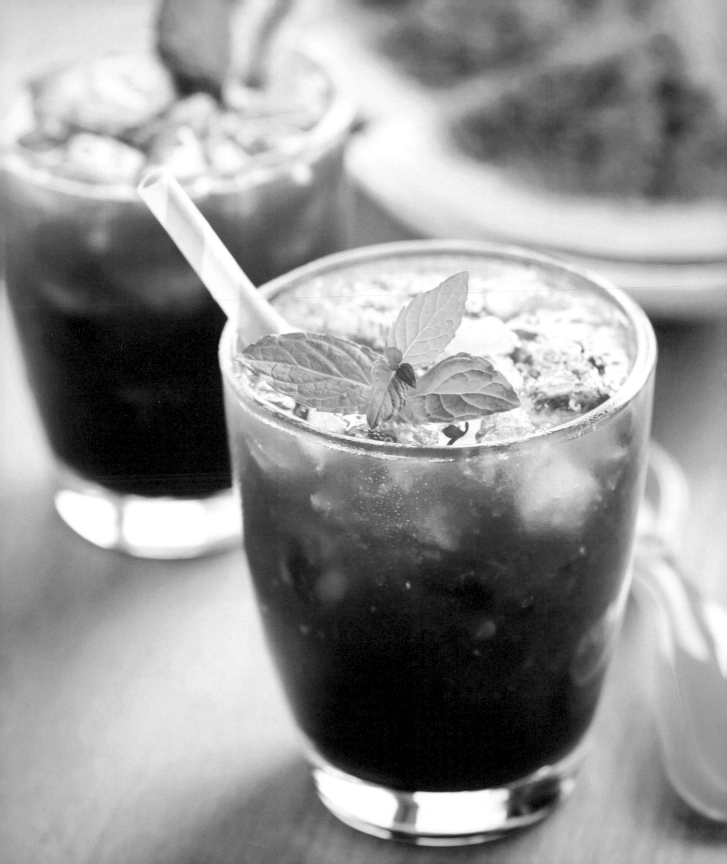

Watermelon-Cucumber Cooler

Perfect for hot summer days, this super-hydrating, cool, and refreshing juice is full of antioxidants and vitamins A and C. It's so delicious, it might just become your go-to juice of the summer!

1 cup watermelon, cut into chunks
½ cup honeydew melon, cut into chunks
½ cucumber
¼ lime

Combine all ingredients in a juicer. Pour juice into a glass or over ice and drink immediately.

> **Honeydew melon has a high water content of about 90 percent, which means it's great for keeping you well hydrated.**

Try this: For an extra-refreshing juice, add 8–10 mint leaves before juicing.

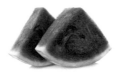

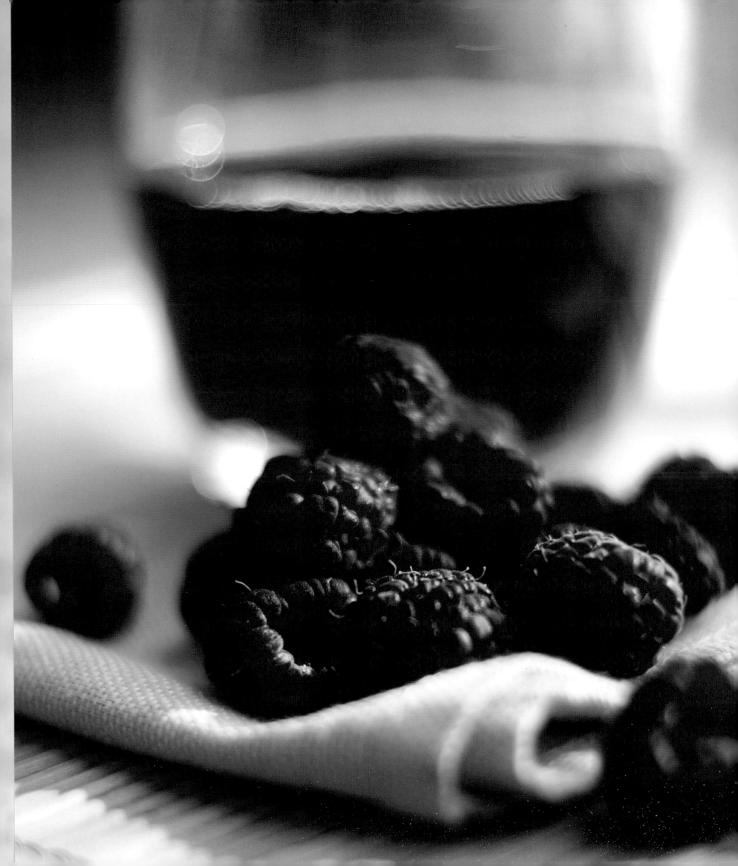

Pineapple-Strawberry Juice

Pineapple, strawberry, and apple—all of my favorites in one juice! This juice tastes a little tropical and a whole lot sweet!

1.5 cup of fresh pineapple, cut into chunks
1.5 cup strawberries
1 apple

Combine all ingredients in a juicer. Pour juice into a glass or over ice and drink immediately.

Try this: For a hint of sweet citrus, replace apple with a tangerine or orange.

 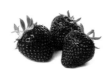

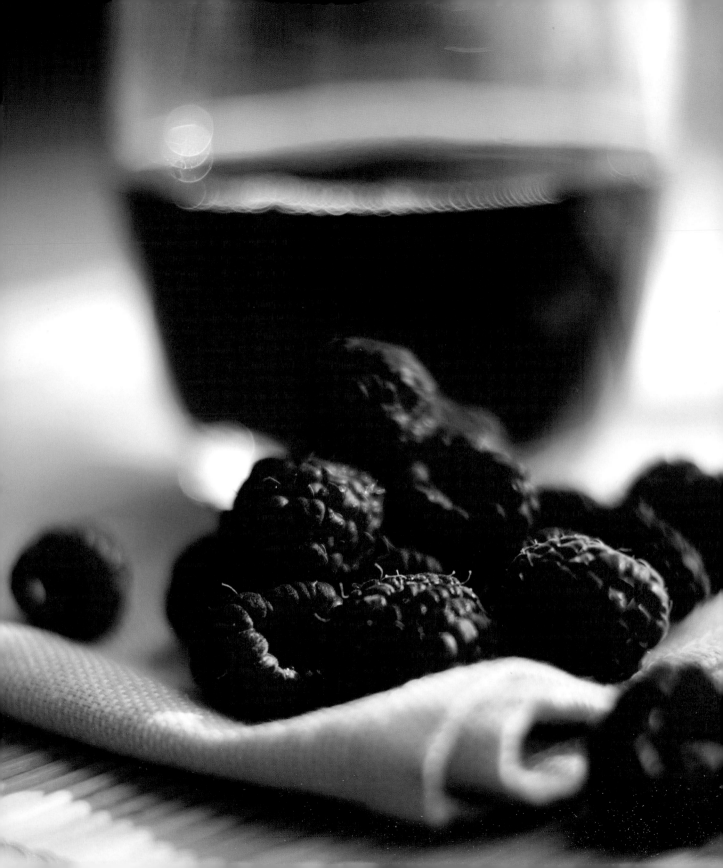

Berry Blend

Here's a sweet berry blend for you! Pick your choice of fresh berries and then juice them with cantaloupe and red or green grapes. You're definitely in for a treat!

2 cups fresh mixed berries (blueberries, blackberries, or raspberries)

1 cup cantaloupe, cut into chunks

½ cup green or red grapes

Combine all ingredients in a juicer. Pour juice into a glass or over ice and drink immediately.

Try this: Replace cantaloupe with 1 cup of watermelon.

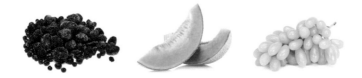

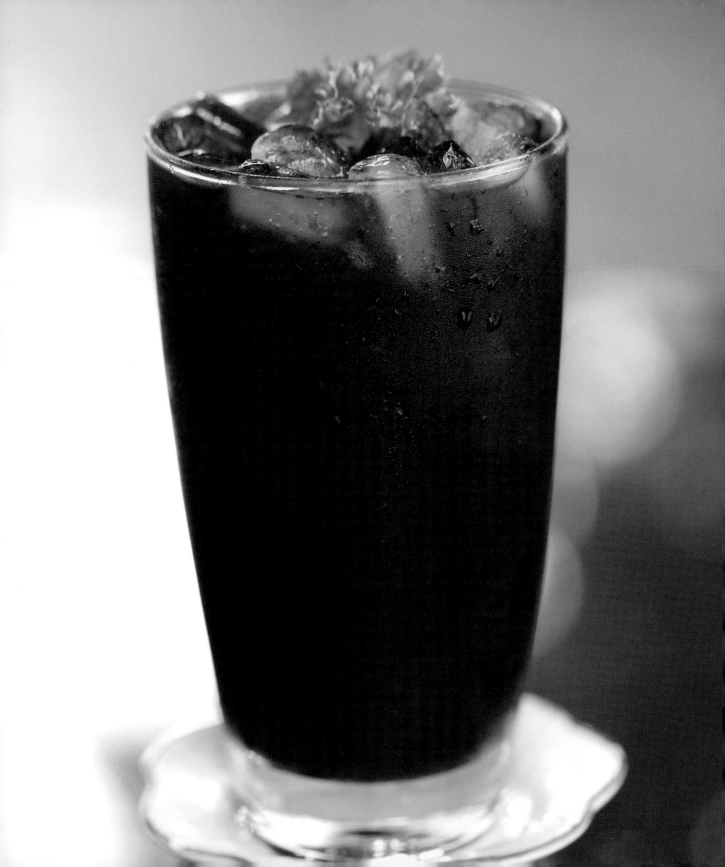

Plum-Berry Juice

Plums and blueberries—what a delicious combination! When mixed with apple and cucumber, you'll enjoy an especially sweet and refreshing juice.

3 plums, pitted
1 cup blueberries
1 apple
½ cucumber

Combine all ingredients in a juicer. Pour juice into a glass or over ice and drink immediately.

Plums are a good source of potassium, a mineral that helps manage high blood pressure and reduces the risk of stroke. In addition, plums contain lutein, an antioxidant that may help promote skin and eye health.

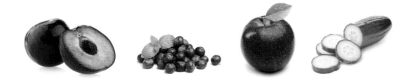

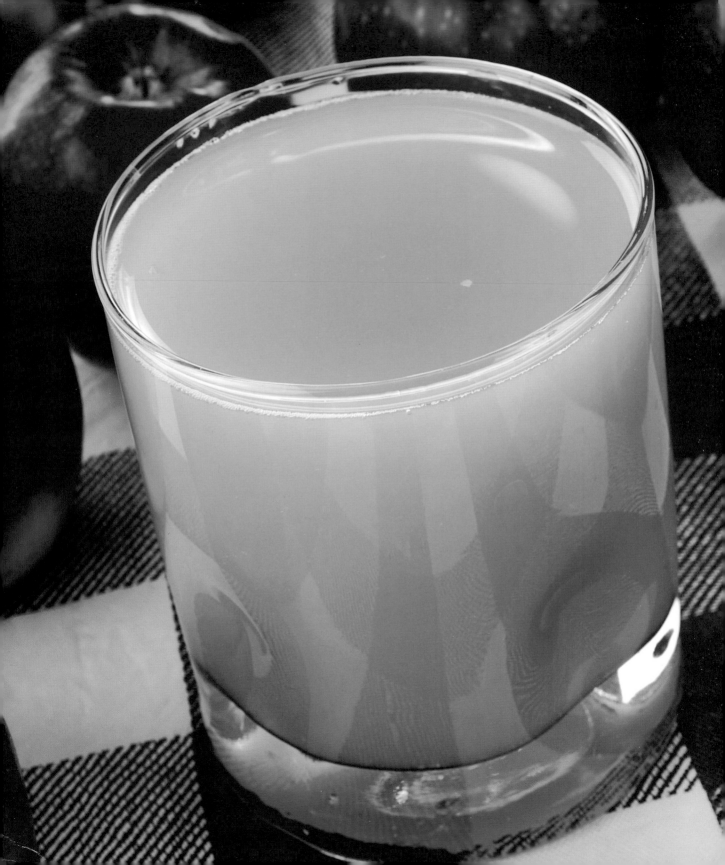

Sour Apple Juice

This isn't your normal glass of apple juice! This one is tangy and sour, thanks to some fresh lemon and ginger.

2 Granny Smith apples
1 cup green grapes
½ lemon
Fresh ginger root to taste (optional)

Combine all ingredients in a juicer. Pour juice into a glass or over ice and drink immediately.

"How do you like them apples?"
—MATT DAMON IN *GOOD WILL HUNTING*

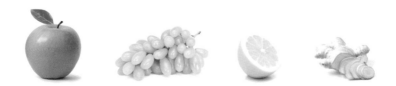

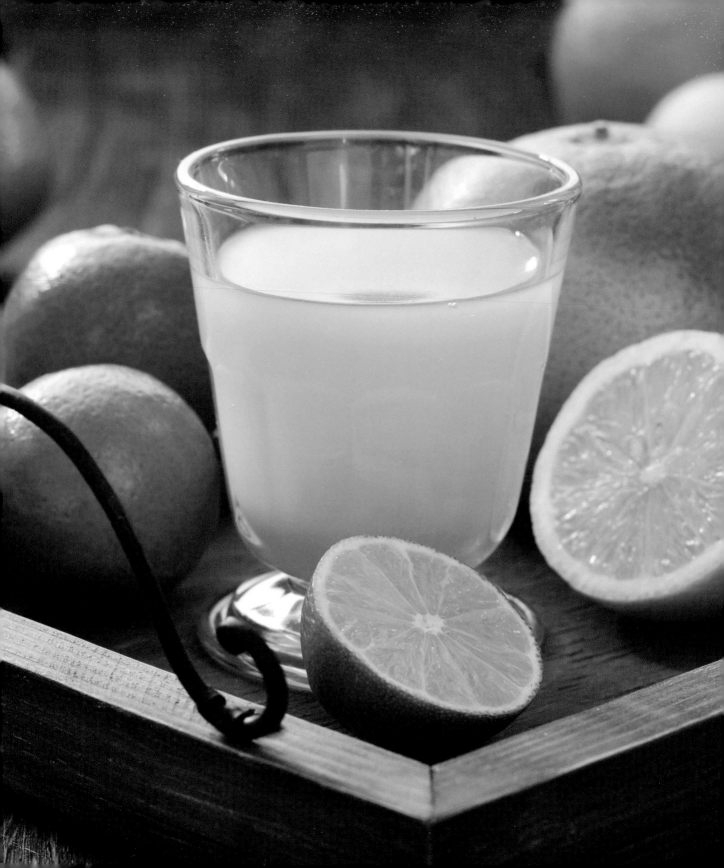

Vitamin C Blend

Vitamin C to the rescue! Feeling a little sluggish and need a natural boost? This juice is for you. Loaded with all sorts of vitamin-rich ingredients, this citrus blend tastes great and provides your daily dose of vitamin C.

2 oranges

2 kiwis, peeled

½ pink grapefruit, peeled and sectioned

¼ lime

¼ lemon

Fresh ginger root to taste (optional)

Combine all ingredients in a juicer. Pour juice into a glass or over ice and drink immediately.

Try this: After juicing ingredients, add ½ tsp of cinnamon.

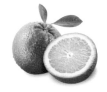

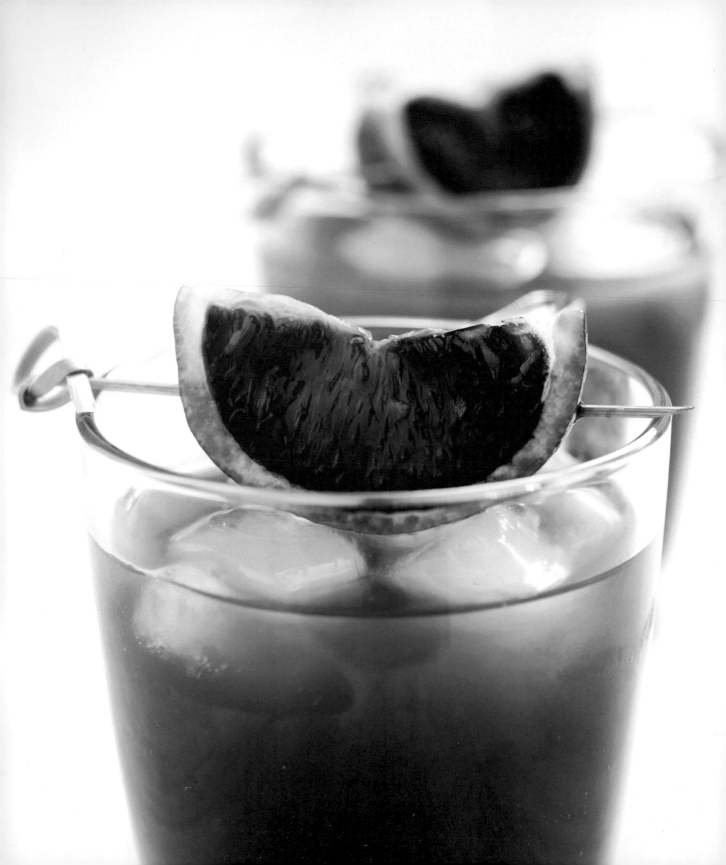

Strawberry Fields

Fresh strawberry juice? You bet! This one is blended with cucumber, orange, and carrots for a delicious blend of fruits veggies.

2 cups strawberries, stems removed
½ cucumber
1 blood orange, peeled and sectioned
2 carrots

Combine all ingredients in a juicer. Pour juice into a glass or over ice, garnish with a skewered section of blood orange if you'd like, and drink immediately.

Who knew? Strawberries have more vitamin C than an orange!

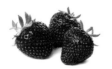 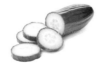 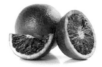 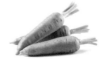

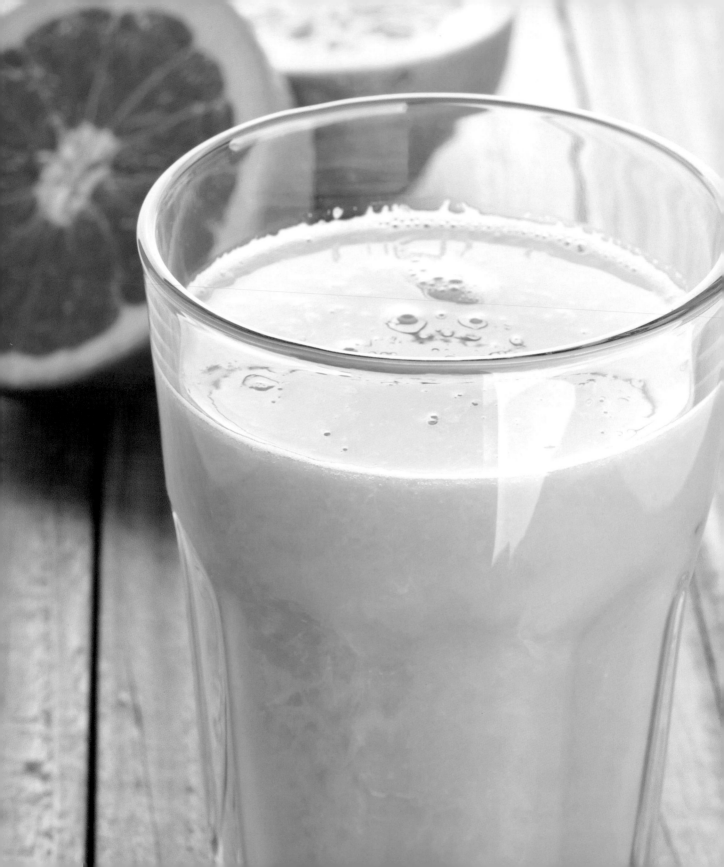

Orange Crush

This isn't your usual orange juice! Crisp apple, sweet cantaloupe, and fresh lemon combine for a flavor combination that will ignite your senses.

2 oranges
1 apple
1 cup cantaloupe, cut into chunks
¼ lemon

Combine all ingredients in a juicer. Pour juice into a glass or over ice and drink immediately.

Try this: For a juicy zing, add fresh ginger root before juicing.

 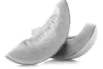 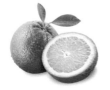

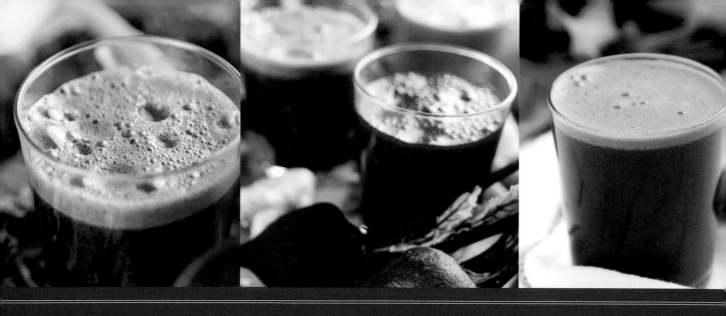

Chapter 10

Vegetable Juice Blends

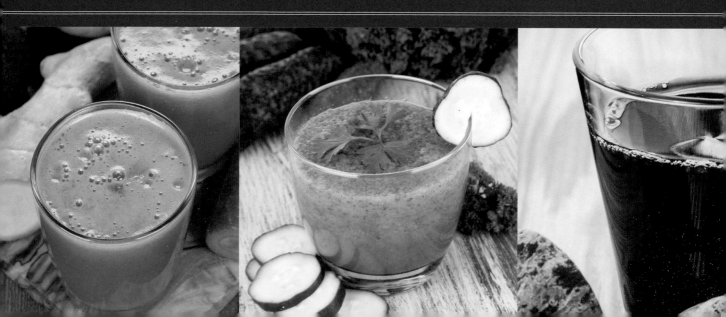

*I*f you're falling short on your daily intake of fresh vegetables, these juice blends are for you! Some of these juices have a half-dozen different veggie varieties in them. How's that for drinking the rainbow? Freshly pressed juice makes it easy to get a plethora of vitamins and minerals in your diet.

The majority of these vegetable juice blends tend to have an earthy, sometimes bitter flavor. You might love how these different vegetable tastes meld together, but if they're too strong for you, try diluting the juice with water or mellowing out the flavor by juicing an apple, pear, or cucumber along with the other ingredients. There's no wrong way to make juice. In fact, the only right way to make it is when you love the taste. Don't be afraid to experiment.

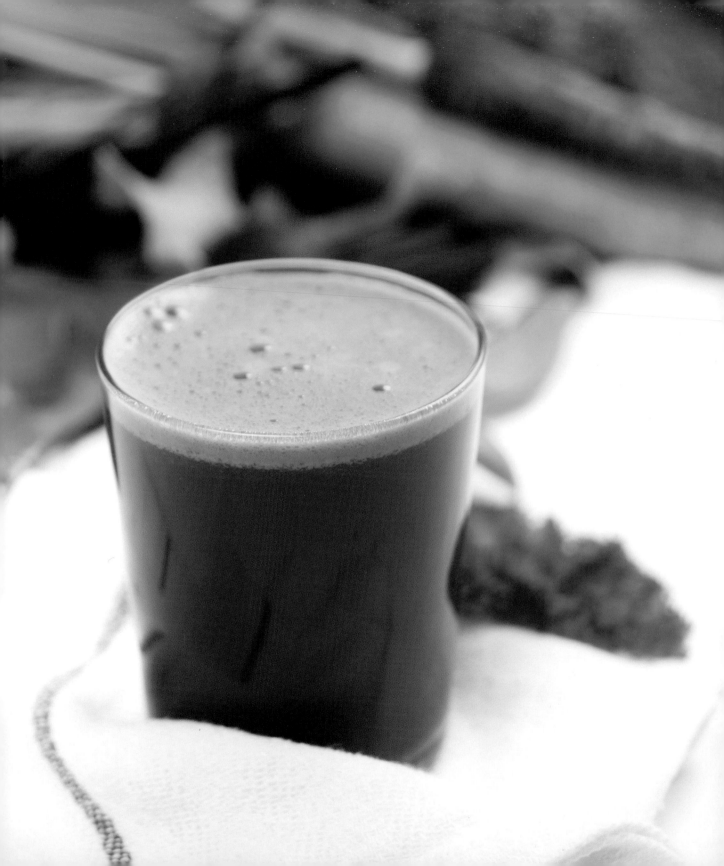

Spicy Mustard Blend

If you like a little kick with your vegetable juice, you need to try this blend made with mustard greens and jalapeño. It's a juice that will bite you back!

4 ounces mustard greens

1 medium tomato

2 carrots

4 celery stalks

½ lemon

½ jalapeño pepper (remove the seeds to make it less spicy)

Put ingredients into a juicer, alternating greens with chunked fruits and veggies. Pour into a glass and drink immediately.

Try this: For a less intense flavor, try fresh spinach, kale, or dandelion greens instead of mustard greens.

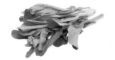 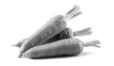   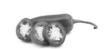

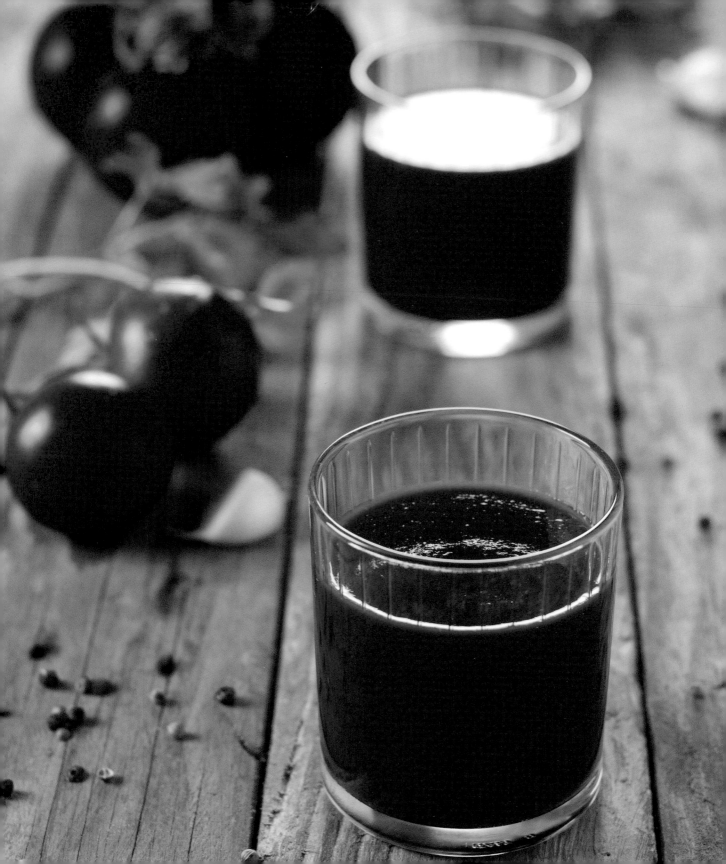

Very Veggie Juice

Start your day on the right foot with this winning combination of vegetables. You'll get a whole slew of nutrients in each sip.

---

3 medium tomatoes

2 carrots

2 celery stalks

½ lemon

1 clove of garlic, peeled

1 piece of horseradish to taste (optional)

Sea salt to taste (optional)

Combine all ingredients in a juicer. Pour juice into a glass or over ice and drink immediately.

Try this: For an extra-spicy vegetable juice, add ½ jalapeño pepper before juicing.

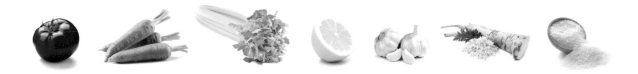

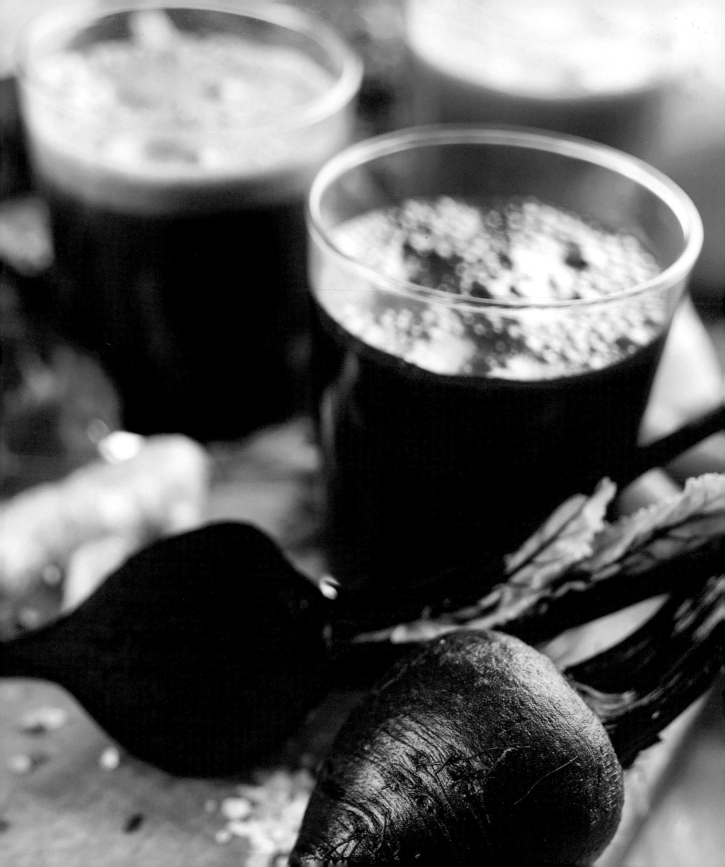

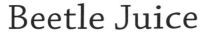

Beetle Juice

You'll love how you feel after drinking it this beet-based juice, loaded with essential vitamins and nutrients.

4 ounces Swiss chard (or spinach)

1 apple

2 beets

2 celery stalks

½ lemon (optional)

Freshly ground pepper to taste (optional)

Put ingredients into a juicer, alternating greens with chunked fruits and veggies. Pour into a glass and drink immediately.

Try this: Add a generous amount of fresh ginger root before juicing.

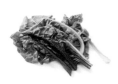 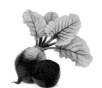

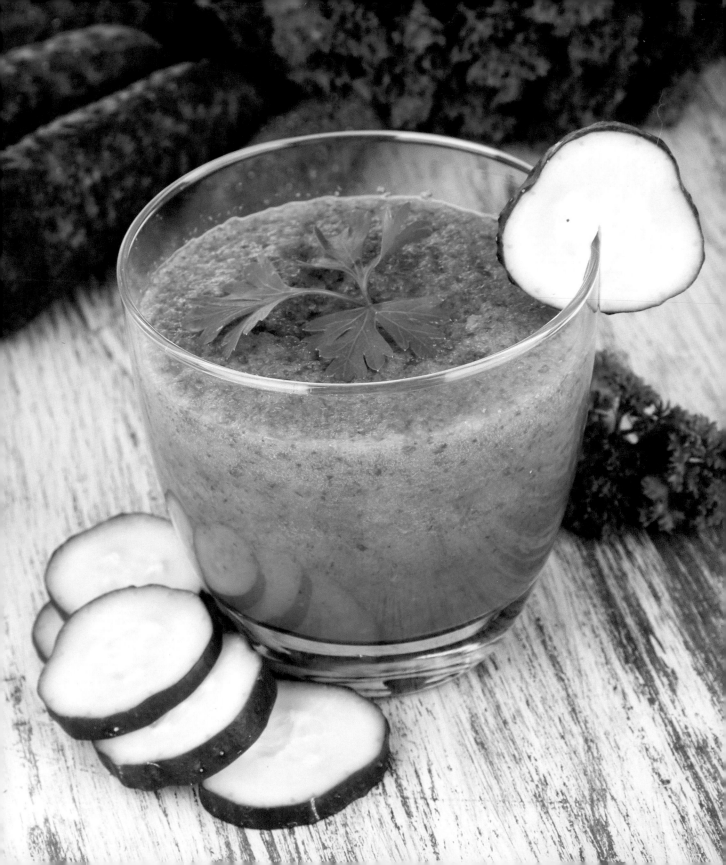

Parsley Lovers' Juice

Do you love the bold, peppery flavor of fresh parsley? If so, this juice is for you. Loaded with a ton of vital nutrients, this juice will wow you in more ways than one.

4 ounces dark leafy greens of your choice

1 cucumber

4 celery stalks

½ bunch to 1 bunch of flat leaf parsley

½ lemon (optional)

Put ingredients into a juicer, alternating greens with chunked fruits and veggies. Pour into a glass and drink immediately.

Parsley is rich in energy-producing chlorophyll and helps to build red blood cells, which increases energy levels.

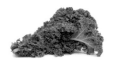 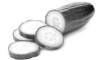 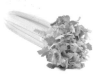

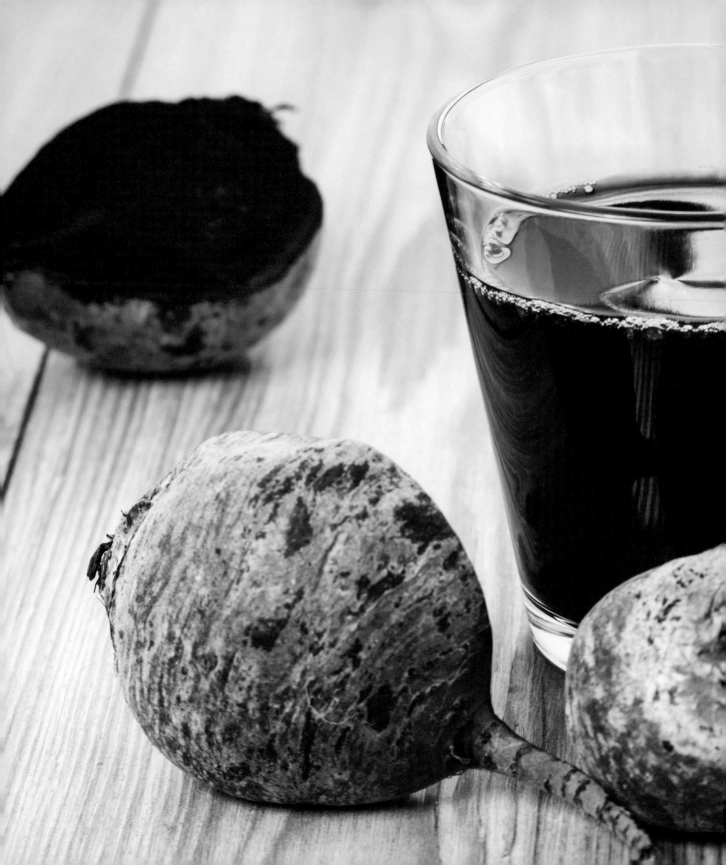

Fearsome Foursome Juice

These four vegetables pack some serious nutrients into one glass of juice. Combine them all together and you'll feel strong and fearless.

2 beets
4 carrots
½ medium sweet potato
1 handful of dark leafy greens of your choice

Combine all ingredients in a juicer. Pour juice into a glass or over ice and drink immediately.

Beets contain a compound that helps fight inflammation and supports the body's natural detox processes. They're also a great source of folic acid as well as vitamin C, which is important for a strong immune system.

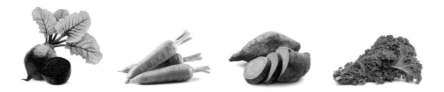

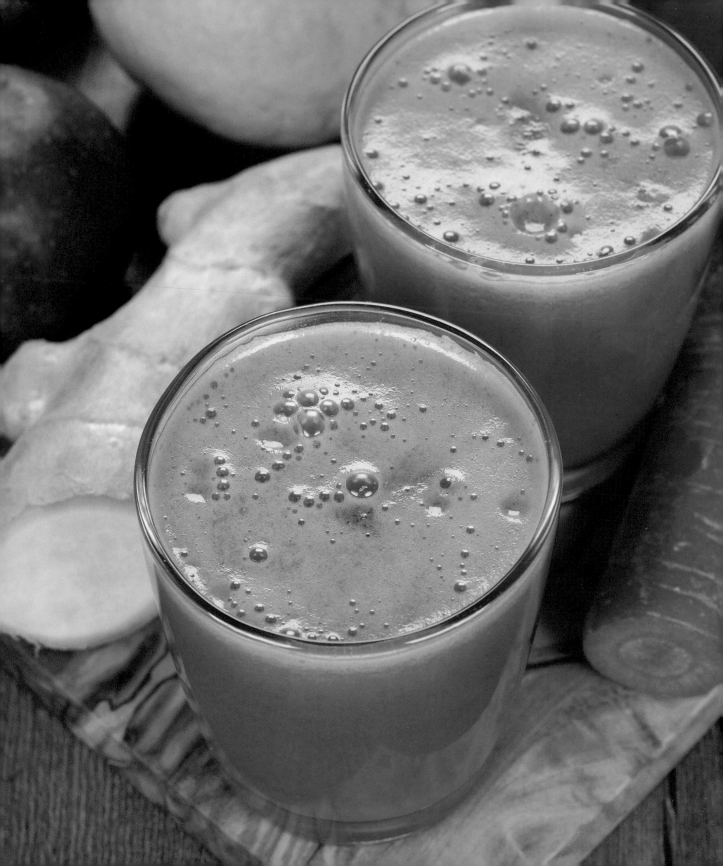

Carrot Juice with a Kick

This isn't your regular glass of carrot juice! Thanks to apple, lemon, and ginger, this one has a little sweet, a little sour, and a whole lot of zip.

6–8 carrots
1 apple
½ lemon
Fresh ginger root to taste

Combine all ingredients in a juicer. Pour juice into a glass or over ice and drink immediately.

> Carrots provide your body with vitamin A as well as a host of other powerful health benefits, including healthy beautiful skin, cancer prevention, and anti-aging properties.

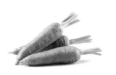

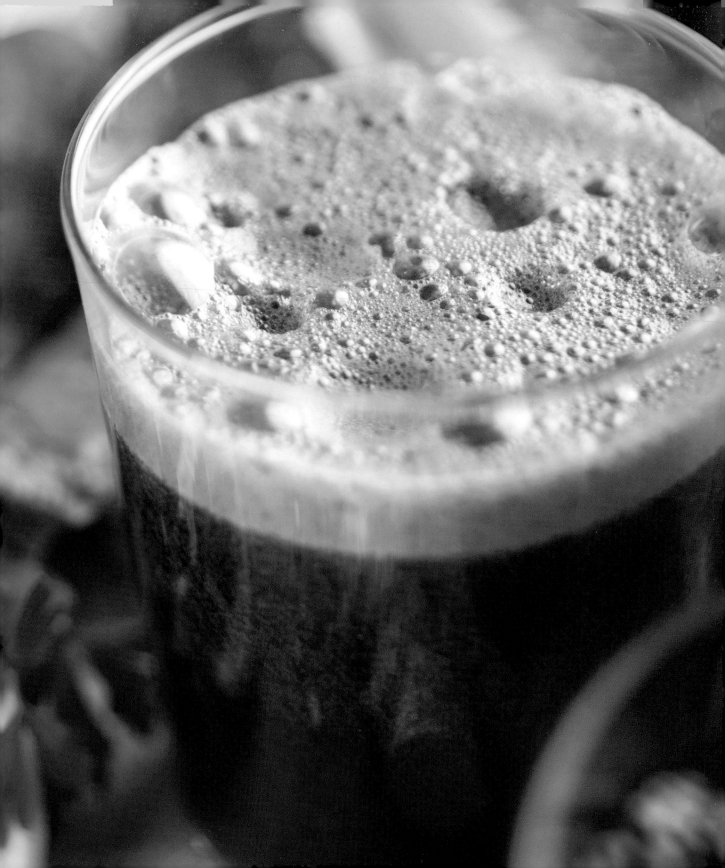

Rainbow Bright Juice

Red, orange, yellow, and green—the colors in these ingredients will brighten up your day and start it off on the right foot.

4 ounces kale (or spinach)

2 cups pineapple, cut into chunks

2 carrots

1 beet

½ lemon (optional)

Fresh mint to taste (optional)

Put ingredients into a juicer, alternating greens with chunked fruits and veggies. Pour into a glass and drink immediately.

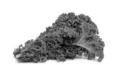 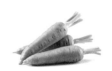

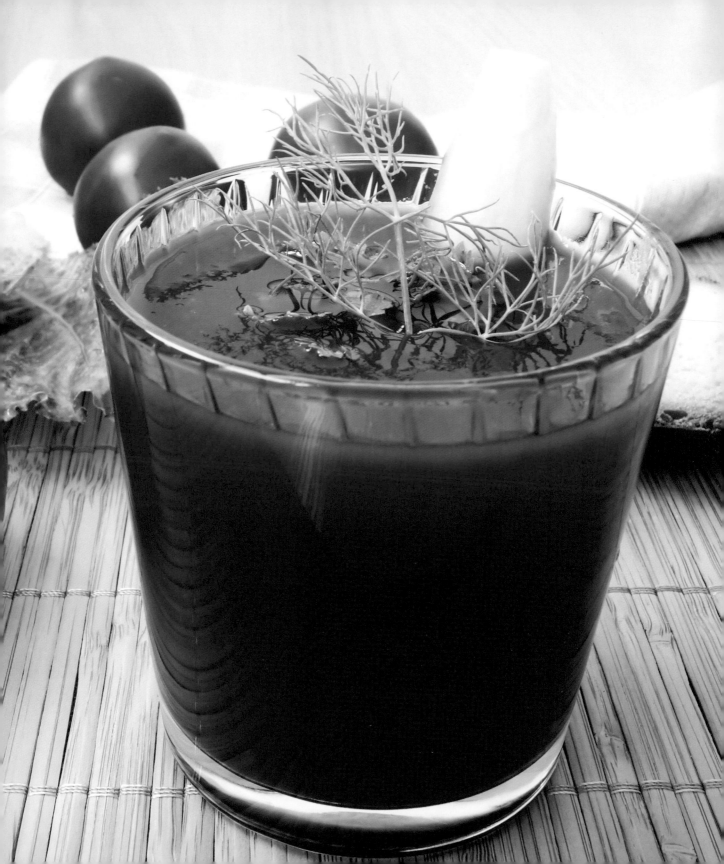

Tomato-Dill Juice

Fresh dill complements tomato so well in this juice. Add a touch of sea salt and freshly ground pepper for a savory juice full of flavor.

4 tomatoes

½ cucumber

1 bunch of dill

Sea salt and pepper to taste

Combine all ingredients in a juicer. Pour juice into a glass or over ice and drink immediately.

Who knew? Chew fresh dill to help alleviate halitosis (bad breath)!

 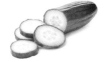

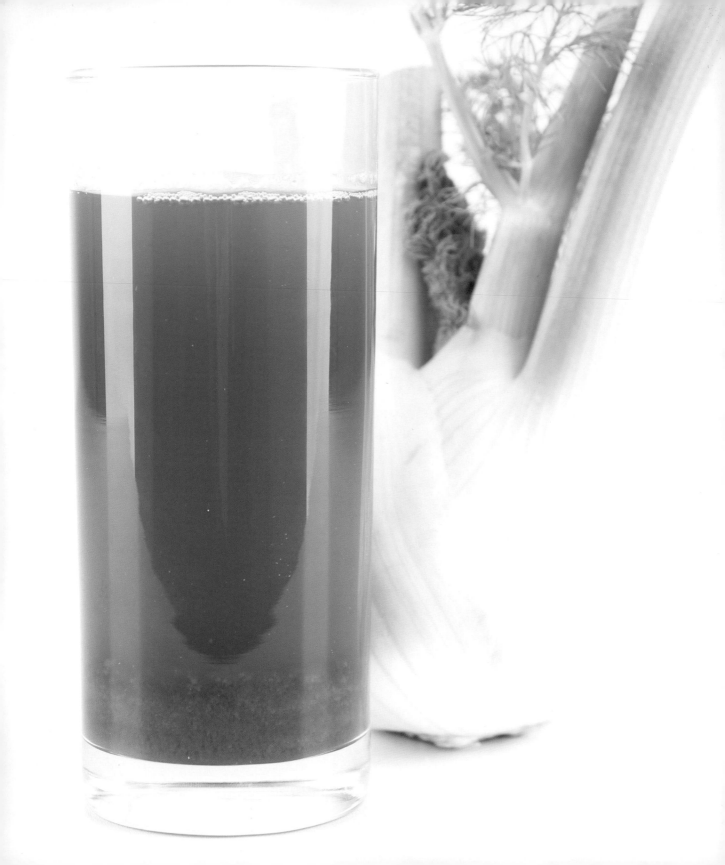

Kale-Fennel-Carrot Juice

Looking to try a new flavor in your juice? Try fresh fennel. It adds a fun, little zing to fresh juice. This juice includes nutrient-rich kale, carrots, and cucumber for a well-rounded and balanced juice.

4 ounces kale

4 carrots

1 cucumber

½ fennel bulb

Put ingredients into a juicer, alternating greens with chunked fruits and veggies. Pour into a glass and drink immediately.

Fennel was Thomas Jefferson's favorite vegetable.

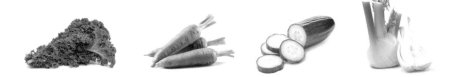

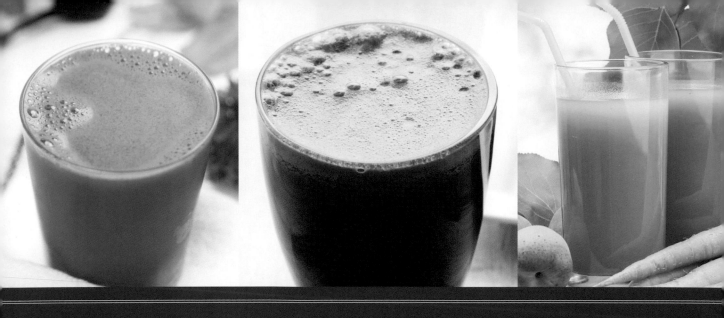

Chapter 11

Energizing Juices

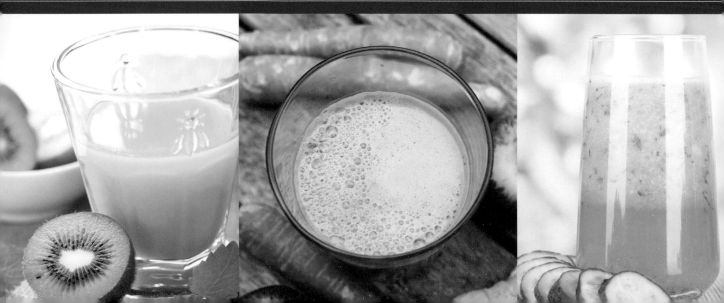

*A*re you dragging today? Lacking focus? Feel like taking a nap? Instead of reaching for a cup of coffee or brownie—both of which give you a temporary jolt of energy—try one of these energy-boosting juices. Drinking caffeine or eating a sweet treat may help you feel better quickly, but it's only temporary. The caffeine or sugar high usually wears off in an hour or so, which puts you right back where you started (and possibly feeling worse than before).

The recipes in this chapter are a natural remedy to help combat that sluggish feeling. They're filled with ingredients that will naturally boost your energy and get you going. Drink them first thing in the morning or in the afternoon to prevent that post-lunch slump.

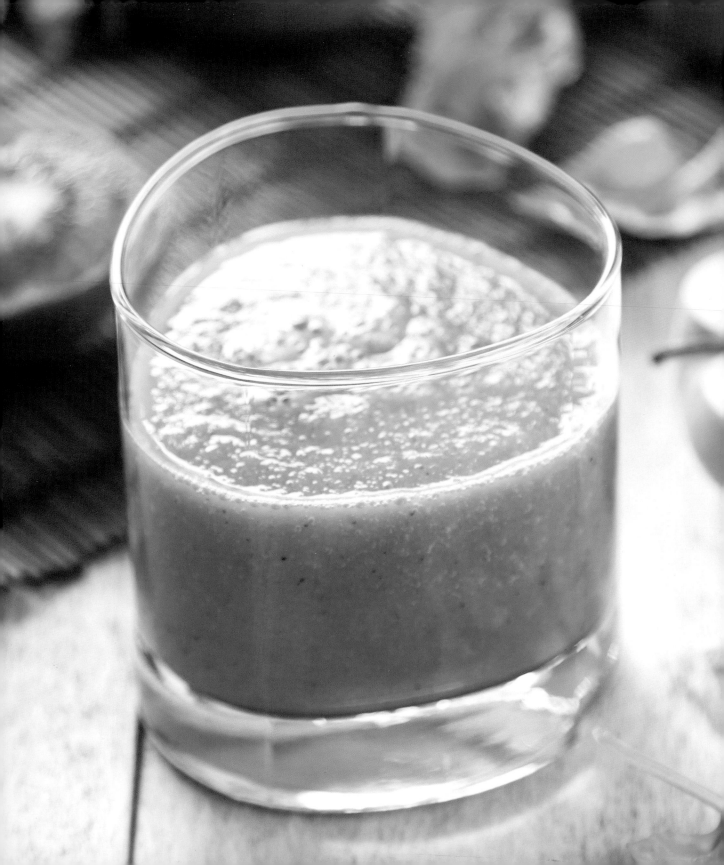

Pear-y Refreshing Juice

If your body is dehydrated, you might feel like you're dragging a little bit. Sip this slightly sweet and refreshing juice to for a boost of hydration and energy!

4 ounces baby spinach

2 pears

1 kiwi, peeled

½ cucumber

Put ingredients into a juicer, alternating greens with chunked fruits and veggies. Pour into a glass and drink immediately.

Try this: For an even more refreshing juice, add 8–10 springs of mint before juicing.

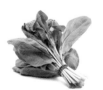

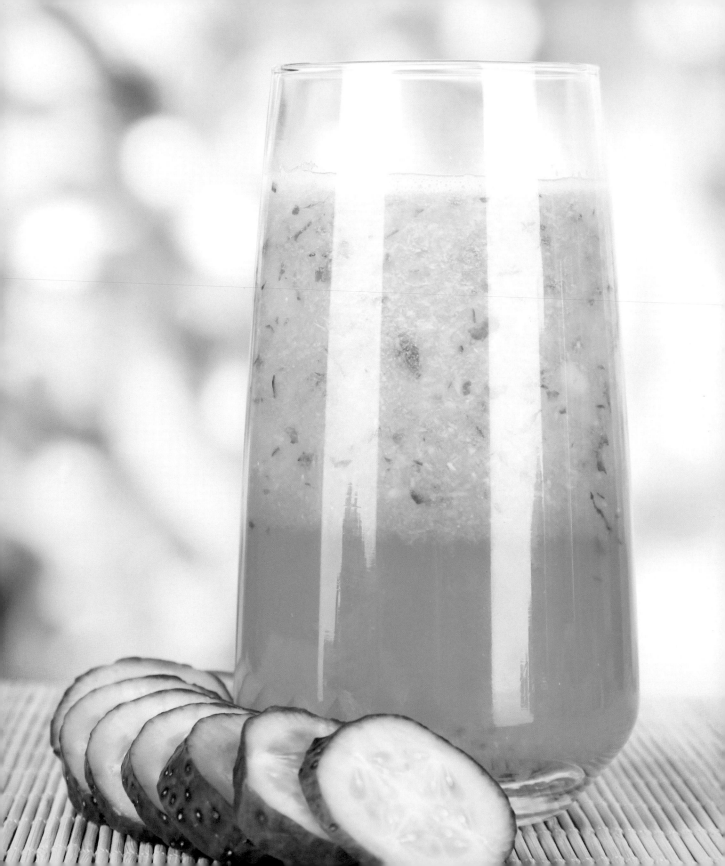

Cucumber Refresher

Cucumber, kiwi, and mint combine for this simple, sweet, and refreshing favorite. Cucumber is great for hydration, so you can drink this juice all day long!

2 cucumbers
2 kiwis, peeled
8–10 leaves of fresh mint

Combine all ingredients in a juicer. Pour juice into a glass or over ice and drink immediately.

> Kiwis are the nutrition powerhouse of fruit. A kiwi has about twice as much vitamin C as an orange and the same amount of potassium as a banana but only half the calories.

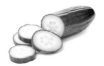

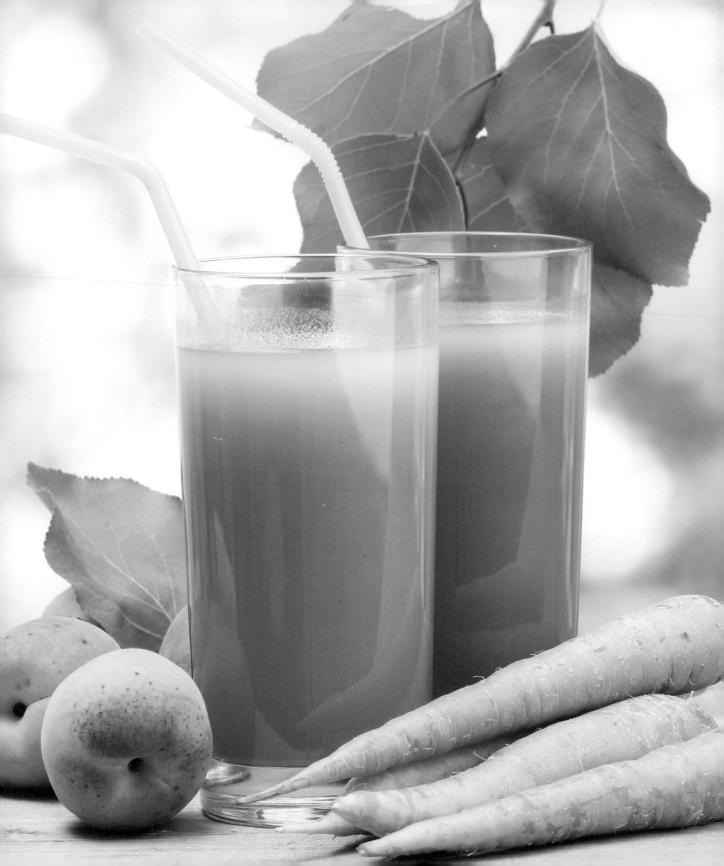

Carrot-Apricot Juice

You may not automatically think to pair apricots and carrots, but you'll be surprised by this delicious blend of flavors.

4 fresh apricots

6 carrots

½ cucumber

Combine all ingredients in a juicer. Pour juice into a glass or over ice and drink immediately.

Try this: For a spicy kick, add freshly grated ginger.

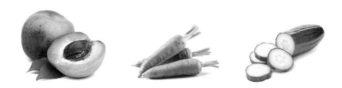

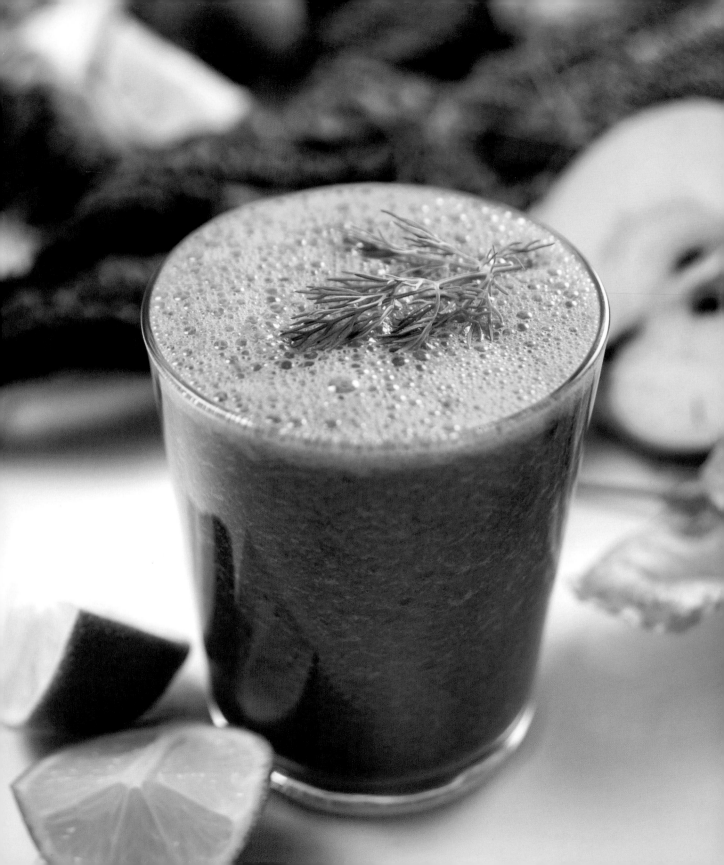

Coconut-Kale-Ginger Juice

Sweet coconut, bitter kale, and refreshing ginger might sound like a unique combination of ingredients, but they meld together so well in this juice. You'll get a natural pick-me-up starting with your very first taste!

4 ounces kale

2 Granny Smith apples

Fresh ginger root to taste

½ cup coconut water

Put ingredients into a juicer, alternating greens with chunked fruits and veggies. Pour into a glass along with the coconut water and drink immediately.

Try this: Not a fan of ginger? Skip it and add 8–10 leaves of fresh mint.

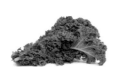

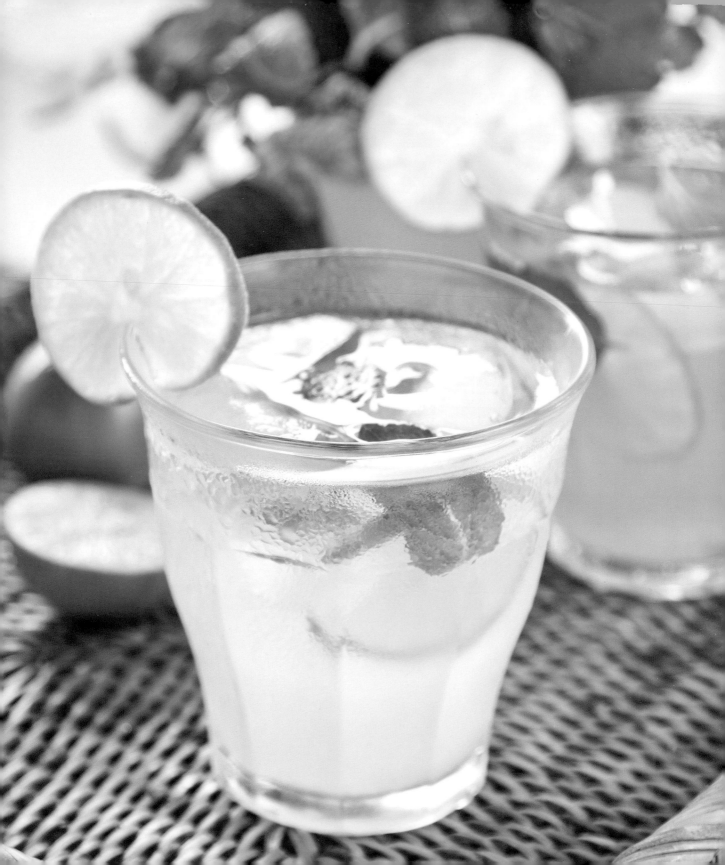

Coconut-Lime Juice

Coconut water is incredibly hydrating, which will give you an instant boost if you're feeling a little parched. Juiced with fresh lime, apple, and spinach, it'll provide your body with a whole host of feel-good nutrients.

1 lime
½ apple
1 cup coconut water
Handful of spinach (optional)

Put solid ingredients into a juicer, alternating greens with chunked fruits and veggies. Combine with the coconut water, pour into a glass, and drink immediately.

> "It is health that is real wealth and not pieces of gold and silver."
>
> —MAHATMA GANDHI

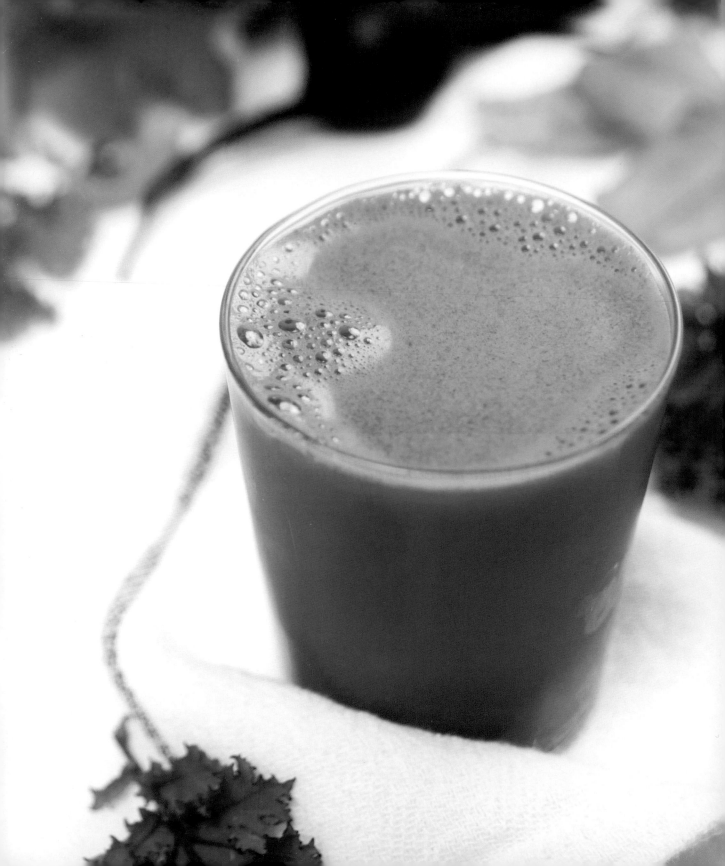

Golden Beet–Citrus Juice

Golden beets tend to have a mellow and earthy taste, so when combined with bold citrus, you'll be pleasantly surprised with how greatly these flavors are enhanced. And, of course, you'll love the eye-catching colors in this juice!

2 small golden beets (or one large)

4 carrots

1 orange, peeled and sectioned

½ apple

Fresh ginger root to taste (optional)

Combine all ingredients in a juicer. Pour juice into a glass or over ice and drink immediately.

> Yellow beets tend to be less sweet and mellower with a less earthy flavor than red beets.

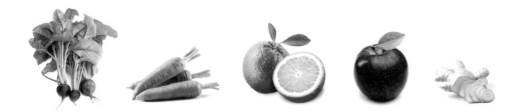

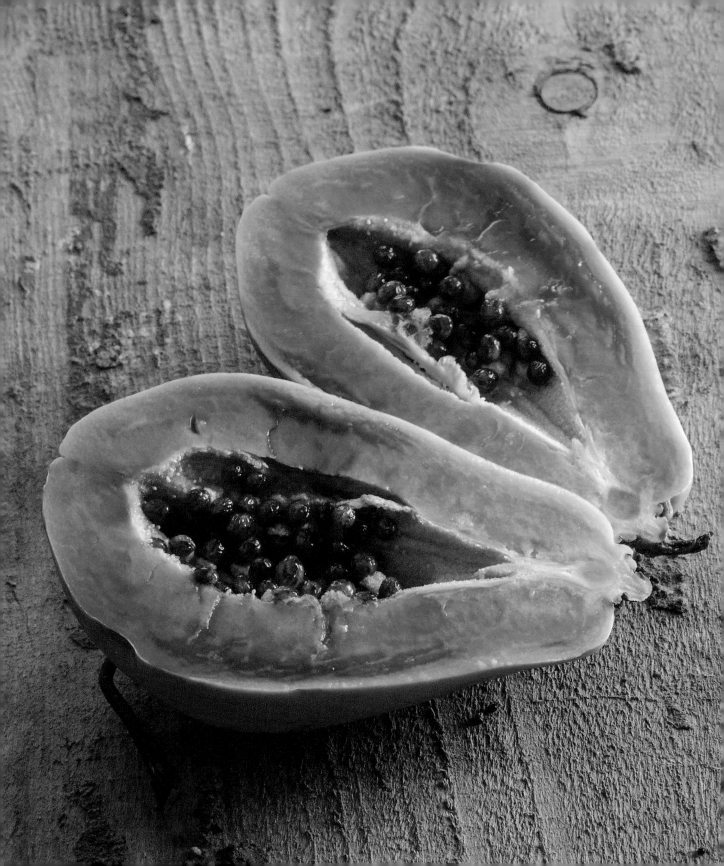

Papaya Pleaser

A small papaya contains about 300 percent of the recommended daily amount of vitamin C. Pineapple, apple, and lemon also contain this immunity-boosting superstar, so you'll definitely get what you need for the day with this juice.

1 papaya, seeded and cut into chunks
1 cup pineapple, cut into chunks
1 apple
½ lemon (optional)

Combine all ingredients in a juicer. Pour juice into a glass or over ice and drink immediately.

When buying papayas, look for ones that are mostly yellow and give slightly to pressure. Avoid the green ones; they'll never properly ripen.

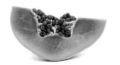

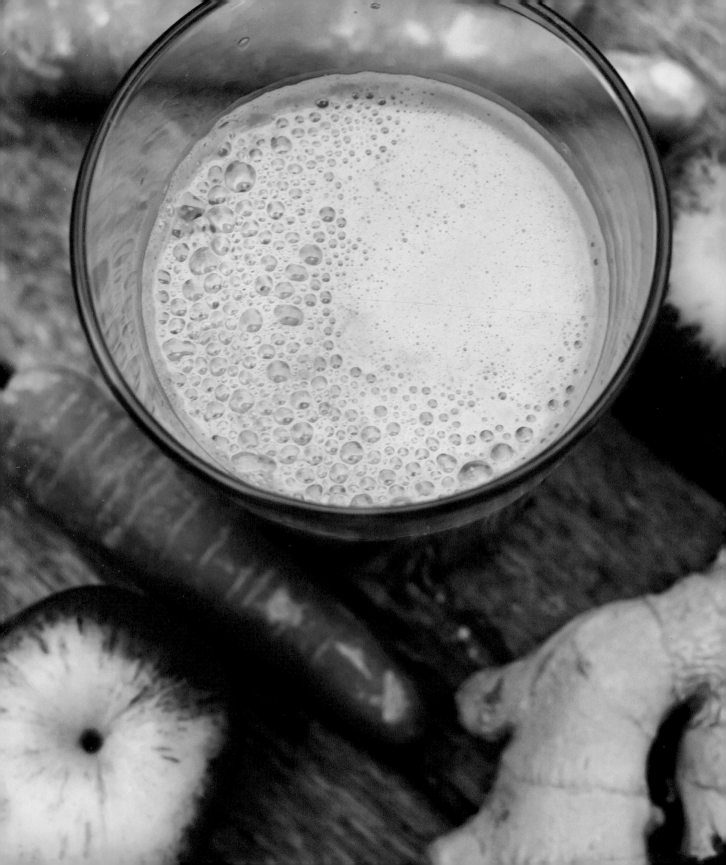

Carrot-Ginger-Apple Juice

This colorful, zesty mixture of carrot, apple, and fresh ginger will wake up your senses and give you an instant, natural lift. Drink this juice whenever you feel the need to be revived.

5–6 carrots

2 apples

Fresh ginger to taste

Combine all ingredients in a juicer. Pour juice into a glass or over ice and drink immediately.

Try this: Omit apples and add one pink grapefruit.

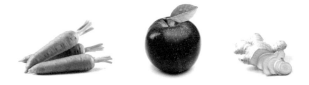

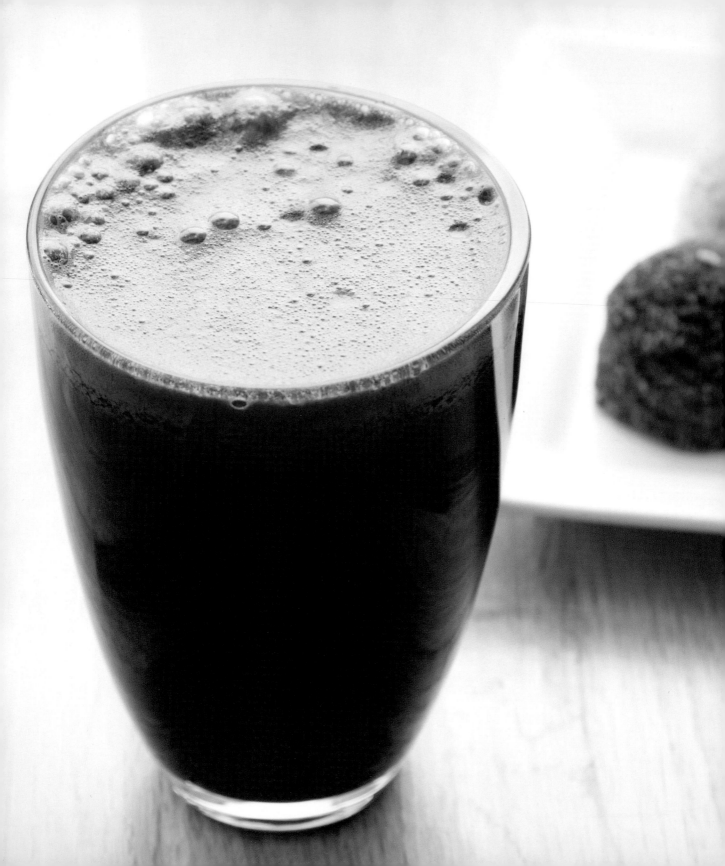

Beet-Apple-Mint Juice

Rich in energy-boosting nutrients, this juice will make you feel full of life. Beets, apple, and mint are an unforgettable combination that will liven your senses.

3 apples
3 beets
8–10 mint leaves

Combine all ingredients in a juicer. Pour juice into a glass or over ice and drink immediately.

Try this: Omit mint and try fresh ginger root instead.

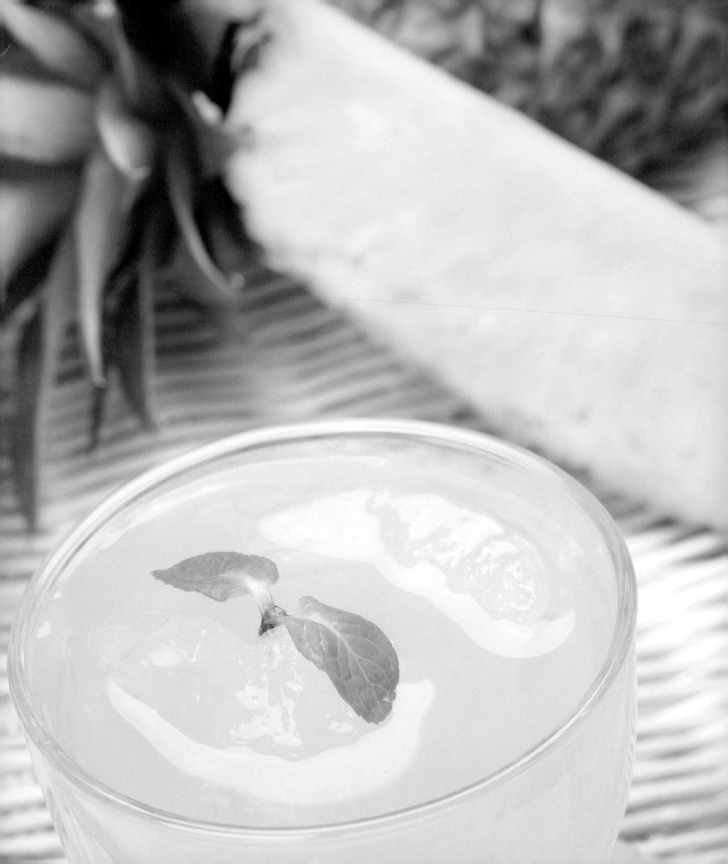

Pineapple Refresher

Drinking a brightly-colored, nutrient-rich glass of juice is a great way to instantly give you a lift, and this juice does just that thanks to citrus fruits, sour apple, and fresh mint. Even your taste buds will be wide awake.

1 Granny Smith apple
3 cups pineapple, cut into chunks
½ lemon (optional)
8–10 mint leaves

Combine all ingredients in a juicer. Pour juice into a glass or over ice and drink immediately.

Try this: Reduce pineapple to 2 cups and add 1 cup of pitted cherries.

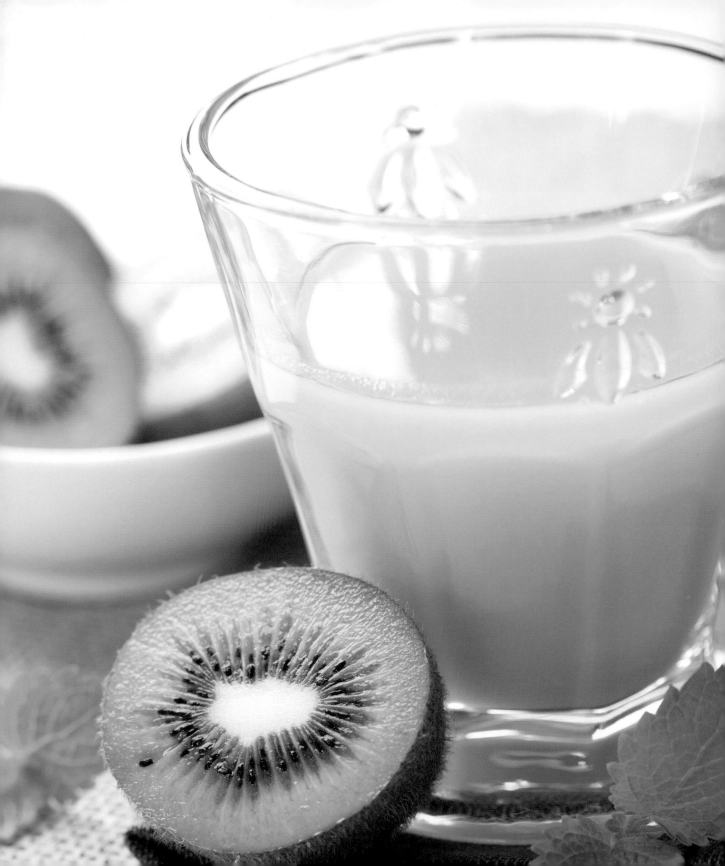

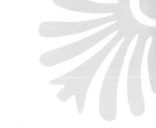

Kiwi Kicker

This juice is loaded with nutrients, so you can start your day off on the right foot or drink it mid-afternoon for a natural energy boost.

1 Granny Smith apple
4 kiwis, peeled
¼ lemon
Fresh ginger root to taste (optional)

Combine all ingredients in a juicer. Pour juice into a glass or serve over ice.

Want a natural boost? Kiwis are rich in magnesium, a nutrient essential for converting food into energy.

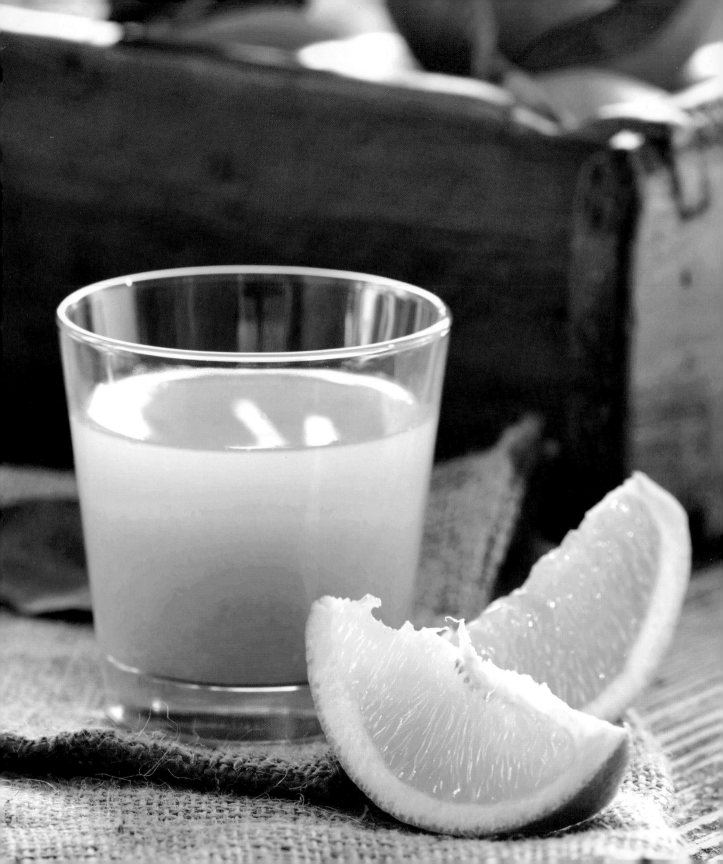

Sunshine Citrus Juice

When you're feeling lethargic and low on energy, skip the energy drink and reach for this sweet citrus blend. Instead of a quick boost that will leave you crashing sooner than later, this juice will give you long-lasting energy.

2 oranges, peeled and sectioned

2 apples

1 sweet potato

Combine all ingredients in a juice. Pour juice into a glass or over ice and drink immediately.

Try this: For a milky alternative, add ¼ to ½ cups of almond milk after juicing the other ingredients. Stir and enjoy.

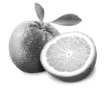

Index

About the Author

Like most brides-to-be, Tina Haupert wanted to look her best on her wedding day. After using an online calorie and exercise tracker and reading food blogs to shape up, Tina was inspired to start her own low-stress nutrition blog, Carrots 'N' Cake.

Since then, Tina's lifestyle blog has become one of the most visited on the Internet. She continues to be super-passionate about keeping a balance—having fun, staying fit, and watching her weight—and sharing her recipes and workouts with her fans.

Tina is a weekly contributor to Health.com as well as an ambassador for various brands, including The Laughing Cow and Reebok. Her first book, *Carrots 'N' Cake: Healthy Living One Carrot and Cupcake at a Time,* shows readers how they can drop the pounds—and keep them off—by adopting eating habits that are healthy, balanced, and above all, livable.

Tina's work has been published or quoted in numerous publications, including *The Boston Globe, Boston Magazine, Health, Woman's Day, Shape, Fitness, Glamour, People,* and *InStyle.*

Tina lives in Weymouth, Massachusetts, with her husband Mal, and adorable pug Murphy. She is expecting her first child this year.

About Cider Mill Press
Book Publishers

Good ideas ripen with time. From seed to harvest, Cider Mill Press brings fine reading, information, and entertainment together between the covers of its creatively crafted books. Our Cider Mill bears fruit twice a year, publishing a new crop of titles each spring and fall.

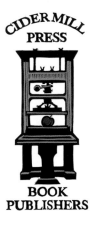

Visit us on the Web at
www.cidermillpress.com
or write to us at
12 Spring Street
PO Box 454
Kennebunkport, Maine 04046